GENE MUTATIONS

CAUSES AND EFFECTS

GENETICS – RESEARCH AND ISSUES

Additional books and e-books in this series can be found on Nova's
website under the Series tab.

GENETICS – RESEARCH AND ISSUES

GENE MUTATIONS

CAUSES AND EFFECTS

HELENA M. CHRISTOFFERSEN
EDITOR

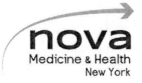

nova
Medicine & Health
New York

NOTICE TO THE READER

Library of Congress Cataloging-in-Publication Data

ISBN: 978-1-53616-984-3

Published by Nova Science Publishers, Inc. † *New York*

CONTENTS

PREFACE

A gene is a DNA sequence that can be transcribed into an RNA molecule and transferred to offspring organisms. Changes in DNA sequences that determine the structure and function of a gene are called mutations. Gene Mutations: Causes and Effects opens by exploring the physical, chemical, and biological agents that cause mutations interact with DNA, leading to genetic instability.

Recent advances in next-generation sequencing have led to the discovery of new causative genes or those mutations. The authors describe the phenotypes and gene mutations, discussing genotype-phenotype correlations compared with previous reports.

Lastly, one study analyses all conflicting data concerning the amplification of the ESR1 gene, particularly its ambiguous prevalence in both untreated tumors and tumors either responsive or unresponsive to antiestrogen therapy.

Chapter 1 - The DNA molecule is a very stable molecule, responsible for the execution of all biological functions in our cells. Thanks to this stability, genetic information is transmitted to the offspring in a correct way for generations. Gene is a DNA sequence that can be transcribed into an RNA molecule and transferred to offspring organisms. Changes in DNA sequences that determine the structure and function of a gene are called mutations. Mutations can be in protein-encoding sequences or in transcription-regulating sequences (promotor, enhancer, silencer, insulator,

UTR, etc.). Physical, chemical, or biological agents that cause mutations interact with DNA, leading to genetic instability. Mutations can be harmful, beneficial or neutral to the organism by causing the DNA sequence to acquire a new function or to lose the function of the gene. Most mutations are known to have deleterious effects and are the source of many diseases and disorders (cancer, hemoglobinopathies, Werner syndrome, Parkinson's disease, Huntington's disease, Xeroderma pigmentosum, etc.). Mutations increase the occurrence of genetic variations in populations and may lead to a stronger adaptation of the organism to the changing environment than others (e.g., the Δ32 mutant in the human CCR5 gene does not catch AIDS). Neutral mutations that do not alter the function of the protein cause polymorphisms by creating silent genetic alterations. These polymorphisms can also give an advantage to living things in the evolutionary process.

Chapter 2 - Hereditary motor neuron diseases can be grouped into three categories. Those with upper motor neuron involvement are called hereditary spastic paraplegias (HSP), those with lower motor neuron involvement are referred to as spinal muscular atrophy (SMA), distal hereditary motor neuropathy (dHMN), Charcot-Marie-Tooth disease (CMT), and those with combined upper and lower motor neuron involvement are designated as familial amyotrophic lateral sclerosis (FALS). They are caused by mutations in the various genes. Recent advances in next-generation sequencing have discovered new causative genes or those mutations. The authors could identify several gene mutations in HSP, CMT, and FALS families using whole-exome or genome sequencing. In this review, the authors described the phenotypes and gene mutations and discussed genotype-phenotype correlations compared with previous reports.

Chapter 3 - The reported amplification of the estrogen receptor alpha gene (*ESR1*) in breast cancers initiated a broad and still ongoing scientific debate on the prevalence and clinical significance of this genetic alteration. The presented study analyses all conflicting data concerning the amplification of *ESR1* gene; its ambiguous prevalence in both untreated tumors and tumors either responsive or unresponsive to antiestrogen therapy. The fact will be highlighted that in healthy breast cells, the dynamism of genome stabilizer machinery may induce *ESR1* amplification when an emergency situation, such as estrogen deficiency requires a rapid compensatory upregulation of estrogen receptor (ER) expression and activation. In contrast, in breast cancer cells, the feedback mechanism between *ESR1* gene and ERs exhibits failures attributed to various alterations of the genome stabilizer circuits. *ESR1* amplification in breast cancer cells may not be expected to show either a direct or indirect correlation with the aggressivity of tumors attributed to various disturbances of their regulatory processes. In antiestrogen treated breast cancers, basal failures of the genomic machinery are exaggerated via the artificial inhibition of the ER activation. The medical blockade of ERs is an emergency state even for tumor cells and a chaotic fight develops between the inhibition of ERs and the compensatory efforts for ER activation. When the medical ER blockade is successful, tumors exhibit unrestrained growth, whilst when the endogenous compensatory actions re-establish ER activation; tumors may show a clinical response. Abundant, reactivated ERs are capable of restoring the altered genomic machinery of tumor cells leading to a self directed apoptotic death. In conclusion, *ESR1* amplification is not an indicator of oncogenic adaptation in tumor cells, and it may not predict either the response or resistance of antiestrogen treated tumors.

In: Gene Mutations: Causes and Effects   ISBN: 978-1-53616-984-3
Editor: Helena M. Christoffersen   © 2020 Nova Science Publishers, Inc.

Chapter 1

TYPES OF GENE MUTATIONS AND THEIR MECHANISMS

Mehmet Buyukleyla[1], Eyyup Rencuzogullari[2], Muhsin Aydin[2] and Mehmet Arslan[3]*

[1]Vocational School of Health Services,
Ardahan University, Ardahan, Turkey
[2]Department of Biology, Faculty of Science and Letters,
Adiyaman University, Adiyaman, Turkey
[3]Department of Nursing, Faculty of Health Sciences,
Ardahan University, Ardahan, Turkey

ABSTRACT

The DNA molecule is a very stable molecule, responsible for the execution of all biological functions in our cells. Thanks to this stability, genetic information is transmitted to the offspring in a correct way for generations. Gene is a DNA sequence that can be transcribed into an RNA molecule and transferred to offspring organisms. Changes in DNA sequences that determine the structure and function of a gene are called mutations. Mutations can be in protein-encoding sequences or in

---

* Corresponding Author's Email: mehmetbuyukleyla@ardahan.edu.tr.

transcription-regulating sequences (promotor, enhancer, silencer, insulator, UTR, etc.). Physical, chemical, or biological agents that cause mutations interact with DNA, leading to genetic instability. Mutations can be harmful, beneficial or neutral to the organism by causing the DNA sequence to acquire a new function or to lose the function of the gene. Most mutations are known to have deleterious effects and are the source of many diseases and disorders (cancer, hemoglobinopathies, Werner syndrome, Parkinson's disease, Huntington's disease, Xeroderma pigmentosum, etc.). Mutations increase the occurrence of genetic variations in populations and may lead to a stronger adaptation of the organism to the changing environment than others (e.g., the Δ32 mutant in the human CCR5 gene does not catch AIDS). Neutral mutations that do not alter the function of the protein cause polymorphisms by creating silent genetic alterations. These polymorphisms can also give an advantage to living things in the evolutionary process.

Keywords: mutation, gene, intron, exon, ORF, mutagen, oncogen

1. INTRODUCTION

When Gregor Mendel published his cross breeding experiments with peas in 1866, the genetic age made a silent start, and until 1900, he maintained his silence and had a pause. Mendel's experiments were also confirmed by Hugo DeVries, Karl Correns, and Errich Von Tschemark in 1900, and since then they have continued to make a big impact in the world of science. The "heredity unit" which was called in Mendel studies was named as "gene" by Walter S. Sutton in 1902. In 1941, George W. Beadle and Edward L. Tatum proposed a gene-an enzyme hypothesis. In 1944, Owald Avery, Colin MacLeod, and Maclyn McCarty discovered that the genetic material was DNA and could be transformed. Morgan, while working with *Drosophila melanogaster*, a fruit fly, noticed that some of the flies had white-eye flies among the most common red-eye (wild-type) flies and called these white-eye flies as mutants. In 1953, James Watson and Francis Crick explained the conformational structure of DNA. Subsequent studies have focused on the study of linking enzymes and proteins to genes, and have tried to find out what changes in DNA structure lead to changes in the phenotype of living things. These researchers started these studies by using organisms with phenotypic differences seen in the population at the beginning, then they accelerated their studies by changing the phenotype of the organism themselves (forming mutant organisms) by using agents that would change the genetic material. Today, it is possible to determine whether there are genotypic differences without waiting for phenotypic differences to be observed. This determination is made on the genetic material, the DNA molecule. For more than 70 years we have known that genetic material is responsible for carrying out cellular functions. The DNA molecule is responsible for the execution of all biological functions in our cells and is a very stable molecule. This stability must be maintained in a normal cell. Due to physical, chemical or biological factors, sometimes stabilization cannot be maintained and stability may vary. Disruption of the genome stability is referred as genomic instability. In such a case, abnormalities in the cell may occur depending on the parts where the change leading to stabilization occurs. For example; O6-methylguanine-DNA methyl transferase (MGMT), which plays an important role in DNA repair mechanism, has a cysteine amino acid that binds the methyl group in the methylated nucleotide to itself (Craig et al., 2010; Alberts et al., 2015). If a mutation occurs to cause another amino acid to replace this cysteine amino acid, the methyl group will not be able to be cleaved from the DNA and a change will occur in the control of gene expression that will result in abnormalities in the cell. Total transcripts in human genome (Protein-coding transcripts, Non-sense mediated decay transcripts, Long non-coding RNA loci transcripts) are estimated to be as much as 208,621. 58,870 genes in these transcripts are protein encoding genes, non-coding RNA genes, pseudogenes, and immunoglobulin/T-cellreceptor gene segments, and there are 24,494 protein-encoding genes (https://omim.org/statistics/entry) within these genes. As of July 8, 2019, 6,452 phenotypes with known molecular basis have been identified and 4,114 of these phenotypes are associated with mutations (https://www.omim.org/statistics/geneMap). As it will be expressed later in the section, in any one of the 208,621 transcripts, there is a possibility that mutations of similar or different forms may occur. When mutations first began to be identified, the focus was primarily on protein-coding sequences. However, studies have begun not only on protein-coding sequences but also on all sequences that affect the functioning of the gene, and work in this area is still ongoing. In fact, various databases have been established in relation to phenotypic changes in individuals due to changes in human gene or extra-genic sequences (http://www.hgvs.org/content/databases-tools).

The genome structure of the living things may change due to mutations in DNA sequences of regulatory gene, operator, promotor, enhancer, insulator, etc. could lead to disruption of their interaction with DNA-protein, RNA-protein, protein-protein, miRNA-RNA, and even protein-other biomolecules, which have important roles in the cellular functions (Allison, 2007; Craig et al., 2010; Weaver, 2011; Pierce, 2012; Li et al., 2019). As a result of the disruption of interactions between these molecules, abnormalities occur in the cell. Therefore, a variety of diseases that can adversely affect the life may occur and may directly affect the viability of the cell. This shows how important it is to maintain genomic completeness.

2. GENE

In this section, it will be more appropriate to define the gene first and explain what sequences are affecting the functioning of the gene. Once the gene and related sequences have been defined, the type of mutations (insertion, deletion, duplication, frameshift mutation, and repeat mutation) occur in the gene sequence or sequences that affect gene functioning will be explained. Next, the causes of mutations and the mechanisms of mutations will be described. At the end of this chapter, the beneficial, harmful, and neutral effects of mutations will be discussed.

The gene is the DNA sequence transcribed to a functional RNA molecule, and this sequence is the basic unit of heredity. While most of the genes of prokaryotic organisms show a continuous structure, the genes in eukaryotic organisms show a discontinuous structure called intergenic region (Craig et al., 2010; Snustad and Simons, 2012; Krebs et al., 2018). Once transcribed, the gene region that will participate in translation to determine the protein sequence and ultimately yield a protein is called the *protein gene*. Genes that carry information of RNA species that will function as RNA when transcribed, but which will not subsequently be translated into proteins, are also referred to as *RNA genes* (Brooker, 2012; Temizkan, 2013). Although the average gene length in humans is between 10-15 kb, the smallest of the genes encoding the protein histone H4 gene is 406 bp, the largest dystrophin gene is 2400 kb (2,400,000 bp) (Brown, 2012). The starting DNA sequence comprising an initiation codon (AUG) and a termination codon (one of the UAA, UAG, and UGA triplets) is called *ORF* (*Open Reading Frame*) (Pierce, 2012). An ORF may not always be translated into a protein sequence, such reading frames are called *URF* (*Unknown Reading Frame*) (Krebs et al., 2018). In an ORF, regions that can be translated into the protein sequence within the DNA sequence are called *exon*, and regions that cannot be translated into the protein sequence are called *introns* (Griffiths et al., 2015; Jorde et al., 2016). So far, 118,412 kinds of proteins have been identified in the human genome (https://www.ncbi.nlm.nih.gov/genome/?term=human+genome). The longest gene of these proteins, the dystrophin gene, has 79 exons and 78 introns (Brooker, 2012). Approximately 50% of mammalian genes have more than 10 introns, some genes have a few exons and some have up to 60 exons (Krebs et al., 2018). A typical eukaryotic gene consists of a promotor, 5'-UTR (leader sequence), exon, intron, and 3'-UTR fragments, the region at which the RNA polymerase and many transcription factors bind on DNA to initiate transcription (Gilbert, 2010). Mutations in exons can alter the sequence of a gene and ultimately affect the structure and function of the protein (Bunz, 2016). A single amino acid change (replacement of leucine to methionine) corresponding to the L868M position in the active site of DNA pol α, a variant of DNA polymerases, leads to prolongation of the primer and addition of inaccurate nucleotides during the replication of DNA (Pavlov et al., 2006). Disulfide bonds in the polypeptide chain have important roles in processes such as protein-protein interaction and protein folding in the cell (Alberts et al., 2015). If a mutation occurs in the DNA sequence in response to the codons of the amino acids in the structure of these polypeptides that allow the formation of disulfide bonds, these interactions will be disrupted (Bunz, 2016). Hot spot mutations occurring in the *HER2* gene serve as *oncogenic drivers* in various types of cancer (Cocco et al., 2019). The product of the first discovered *RAS* gene in tumors is an oncoprotein that is effective in cell growth and cell death in the cell communication pathway (Basu, 2018). In RAS proto-oncogene, as a result of mutations causing codons 12, 13, and 61 to change, proto-oncogen transforms into oncogene and forms cancer (Weinberg, 2014). Although introns are not involved in the protein sequence, they have important functions in gene expression such as the determination of exon-intron boundaries or self-splicing introns in the processing of pre-mRNA (Craig et al., 2010; Weaver, 2011; Temizkan, 2013; Griffiths et al., 2015; Turpenny and Ellard, 2017). Mutations in the exon regions directly affect the sequence of the protein to be synthesized. However, mutations that occur in introns, genes encoding non-coding RNAs, regulatory sequences and sequences constituting recognition sites that play an important role in DNA-RNA and DNA-protein interaction affect gene regulation (Clark, 2005; Pierce, 2012; Jorde et al., 2016; Miesfeld and McEvoy, 2017). In order to achieve the degree of gene expression required by the cell, various intra- and extra-gene sequences (promoter, enhancer, silencer, insulator, UTR, terminator, splice fields, branching point for splicings, etc.) are required (Weaver, 2011; Brooker, 2012; Pierce, 2012; Temizkan, 2013; Watson et al., 2014; Klug et al., 2015). These regulatory sequences are well preserved in the genome (Allison, 2007; Watson et al., 2014; Klug et al., 2015). However, it is also known that approximately 15% of mutations leading to genetic diseases in humans result in abnormal mRNA splicings, and approximately 85% of these splicing mutations alter 5' and 3' splice signals (Klug et al., 2015). There are DNA binding sites on the DNA with specific consensus sequences to which transcription factors can bind to carry out the transcription process (Van Straalen and Roelofs, 2012). A mutation in the regulatory sequences may adversely affect the binding of the transcription factors to the regulatory sequence onto the DNA during a normal transcription process. Mutations in promoter sequences can increase, decrease or stop the level of transcription by altering the binding activity of RNA polymerase to the promoter (Pierce, 2012; Temizkan, 2013). A mutation in the regulator element/operon may impair the ability to regulate gene expression (Pierce, 2012). Mutations in the 5'-UTR/3'-UTR regions may impair the function of the RNA to be translated (Jorde et al., 2016). In order to achieve a proper splice, splice acceptor, splice donor, and branch point consensus sequences are required (Allison, 2007; Bunz, 2016). The mutation in these consensus sequences may alter the processing of the pre-mRNA that will undergo of a splicing (Snustad and Simmons, 2012; Jorde et al., 2016). In the lac operon of *E. coli* from the upstream to the downstream, the CAP site, lac promoter (lacP), operator site (lacO), lacZ (β-galactosidase), lacY (permease), lacA (trans acetylase) and lac terminator sequences can be found (Watson et al., 2014). Before the lac operon, there is the regulatory gene *lacI* (lac repressor) and its *i* promoter series (Dale and Park, 2010; Krebs et al., 2018; Klug et al., 2015). A mutation (*lacI*) in the *lacI* gene encoding a repressor protein may lead to a change in the structure of the repressor protein (Temizkan, 2013; Miesfeld and McEvoy, 2017). Such mutational changes in gene expression can result in 3 different ways. First, the repressor protein whose structure is altered cannot binds to *lacO* and transcription does not occur. Second, the repressor protein, whose mutation has changed in structure, binds to *lacO* and is not separated again. As a result, the lac operon remains continuously open and transcription carry on continuously. Third, there is no change in the repressor protein whose structure has changed as a result of mutation in terms of binding to *lacO* (Dale and Park, 2010; Snustad and Simmons, 2012). In this case, transcription continues normally. As it can be seen, transcription can be affected not only when the mutation occurs in the intra-gene region, but also in the extra-gene region, and preservation of all these regions is extremely important for the function of the gene.

3. MUTATION (TYPES AND CAUSES)

The human genome consists of approximately 3 billion base pairs (3×10^9 bp) and the genome similarity between two unrelated individuals is approximately 99.5% (Nussbaum et al., 2015). This difference in the human genome is due to the fact that genomic stability is not fully preserved in the evolutionary process. It should also be remembered that the presence of crosingover leads to individual differences without deteriorating genome integrity. As previously described, mutations in regulatory sequences such as the structural gene, regulator gene, operator, and promoter seen in the genomes of living things disrupt genomic stability. So, genetic changes in DNA sequences that determine the structure and function of a gene, resulting in complete degradation of the genome, are called mutations. Of course, the mutation does not only occur in DNA genomes, but also in RNA genomes, and the rate of mutations in the RNA molecule is approximately 1000 times higher than in the DNA molecule (Madigan et al., 2012). This explains why RNA viruses evolved rapidly than DNA viruses. Mutational changes can occur at very different levels from the change of a single nucleotide to the loss of an entire chromosome (Allison, 2007). Changes in the structure of the gene (sequence and number of nucleotides) without changing the position of genes are called gene mutations (Temizkan, 2013). Mutational changes in the genome sequence resulting from replication errors or damaged nucleotides can also be triggered by physical, chemical or biological agents (Snustad and Simmons, 2012; Cox et al., 2015). DNA-modifying agents, which may be of exogenous or endogenous origin, can produce approximately 70,000-100,000 molecular lesions per day (Voet et al., 2016; Shanbhag et al., 2018). These agents are able to alter the function of the genomic DNA sequence by causing damage such as base loss, base addition, adduct formation or modification of the base structure through oxidation, DNA crosslink formation, DNA-protein crosslink formation, and strand breaks (Greim and Snyder, 2019). Changes in DNA that make the cell malignant are called *driver mutations* (Schildgen and Schildgen, 2018). In a gene, lack of function (LOF) or gain of function (GOF) results in new alleles/genomic variants (Turpenny and Ellard, 2017; Li et al., 2019). Any mutation from a single nucleotide exchange to the loss of the entire gene can lead to loss of function. However, due to mutations of functional gain, it can lead to abnormal expression of the gene at a different level, place, or time (Klug et al., 2015). As a result of the mutation, protooncogene may turn into oncogene, or mutations in non-coding regions of DNA may lead to disruption of the interaction between transcription factors (TF) and binding regions (TFBS) of transcription factors (Li et al., 2019). In the transcription of a gene, a mutation in the DNA sequence that is the binding site for a repressor or inducing protein can alter the expression of the gene of interest (Clark, 2005). In humans, there are 1639 known TF proteins with at least one DNA binding domain, indicating the importance of errors in TF-TFBS interactions (Gonzalez-Perez et al., 2019). They can lead to the loss of existing TFBS with LOF in the DNA sequence or the formation of a new TFBS with GOF. However, such mutations can lead to changes in the binding sites in DNA, not only of TFs but also of non-coding RNAs (Li et al., 2019). While most LOF mutations behave in recessive manner, most GOF mutations behave in dominant manner (Temizkan, 2013).

In all organisms, a certain number of mutations can occur as a result of cellular functions and environmental interactions. Under normal circumstances, most mutations occur spontaneously due to inevitable errors in DNA replication, repair, and recombination (Kondrashov, 2017). Such mutations are called spontaneous mutations. Cells carrying spontaneous mutations that have harmful effects are rare because they are selected, so it is very difficult to observe spontaneous mutations in a natural population. Mutations induced by agents are much easier to observe.

Spontaneous or induced mutations in DNA are not transmitted to offspring if they occur in somatic cells, but may be passed on to offspring if they occur in germ cells (Nussbaum et al., 2015).

Various databases related to phenotypic changes in humans due to changes intragenic or extragenic sequences (Locus Specific Mutation Databases, Central Mutation Databases, Central Mutation & SNP Databases, National & Ethnic Mutation Databases, Variation Databases, and Other Mutation Databases) have been established (http://www.hgvs.org/content/databases-tools). For example, the Locus Specific Mutation Databases database has been created to give answers to following questions; in which region of the genome do mutations occur and what kind of changes occur within the genome. As of 20.05.2019, 1646 genes with locus-specific mutations have been identified. Eighty five different mutations have been identified in the WRN gene that contains 35 exons encoding a helicase (www.pathology.washington.edu/research/werner/database/). There are 17,289 variant of the DMD gene, our largest gene encoding human dystrophin, has been identified ((https://databeses.lovd.nl/shared/ genes/DMD). As changes in the genome are discovered, data entry is provided to these and similar databases.

3.1. Mutation Types

Mutations are considered in two groups as gene mutations and chromosomal mutations: Mutations affecting a single gene are called gene mutations, and mutations affecting chromosome structure and number are called chromosome mutations (Pierce, 2012). This section will focus only on gene mutations. Gene mutations are also called DNA mutations. Gene mutations are alterations that occur in a DNA sequence from a single nucleotide to a size of approximately 100 kb (Nussbaum et al., 2015). Mutations with deletions or insertions of less than 20 bp are called microdeletion or microinsersion, respectively (Bunz, 2016). There may be different kinds and numbers of mutations within a single gene. For example, a total of 4,266 mutations (560 deletions, 220 duplication, 50 indel, 254 insertions, and 3,212 SNP) have been identified for the neurofibromatosis-associated NF1 gene, and these mutations comprise a 5 Mb change from a single base change (https://www.ncbi.nlm.nih.gov/ clinvar).

Gene mutations can be classified as follows;

- Point Mutations
  - Base substitutions
  - Indel mutations (Insertion or Deletion)
- Duplication
- Repeat expansion
- Frameshift mutations

Point Mutation

The source of point mutations is the errors caused by mismatches of the complementary base in the newly synthesized strand during DNA replication (Brown, 2012). There are two types of point mutations that occur due to replication errors: changes involving insertions and deletions called base substitution and indel.

Base Substitution Mutations

Base substitutions are the replacement of one base pair in the DNA sequence with other base pairs (Dale and Park, 2010). These base changes can take two forms: transitions and transversions. *Transition* is the replacement of one purine in the DNA sequence with another purine ($G \leftrightarrow A$) or another primidine instead of one primidine ($C \leftrightarrow T$). On the other hand, if a primidine replaced with a purine ($C \leftrightarrow A$ or $C \leftrightarrow G$, $T \leftrightarrow A$ or $T \leftrightarrow G$) or a purine substituted with a primidine ($A \leftrightarrow C$ or $A \leftrightarrow T$, $G \leftrightarrow C$ or $G \leftrightarrow T$) is called *transversion* (Table 1) (Allison, 2007; Brooker, 2012; Brown, 2012; Pierce, 2012; Cox et al., 2015; Griffiths, 2015). The occurrence of base substitution in a protein encoding gene results in 3 possible conditions: *Missense mutation*, *nonsense mutation*, and *silent mutation* (Madigan et al., 2012). The possible changes on the UUA codon encoding a single amino acid (leucine) can be caused by only a single nucleotide change, these changes could be seen as follows. UUA codon encoding the leucine could be mutated and transformed into the UUG and CUA codons, these codons (UUG and CUA) still encode the same amino acid (leucine) and this mutation is referred as silent mutation. When the UUA codon is mutated and encoded different amino acid such as AUA (isoleucine), GUA (valine), UUU (phenylalanine), UUC (phenylalanine) and UCA (serine) these mutations are referred as *missense mutation*s. Similarly, when the UAA codon transforms to UGA and UAA, which are stop codons, the mutations are referred as *nonsense mutations* (Dale and Park, 2010). The polypeptide sequence may also be altered as a result of missense and nonsense mutation that occur in the protein coding sequences of DNA. For example, if the AAA codon, which encodes the lysine amino acid at the exon site during transcription, changes to UAA, a stop codon, the polypeptide to be synthesized will remain short and a non-functional polypeptide product may be formed. Such a mutation is called a nonsense mutation (Allison, 2007; Pierce, 2010). Non-sense mutation occurs in humans with Marfan syndrome. In humans with this syndrome, a mutation occurs such that the tyrosine amino acid in position 2113 of the fibrillin 1 (FBN1) gene is transformed into a stop codon (Kumar and Eng, 2015). As a result of this meaningless mutation, the polypeptide to be synthesized will be shorter than the normal one and will not function normally. Another type of mutation that leads to changes in the amino acid sequence in the polypeptide chain through point mutations is missense mutations (Allison, 2007, Pierce, 2010). In such mutations, the amino acid in the polypeptide sequence also changes due to the DNA sequence change. For example, instead of glutamic acid, the 6th amino acid of the β-globin polypeptide chain, valine amino acid is replaced with sickle cell anemia (Jorde et al., 2016). This amino acid change occurs as a result of the transcription of the codon encoding the glutamic acid in the DNA sequence to the codon encoding the valine amino acid (transcription, $CTC \rightarrow CAC$) (Weaver, 2011; Brooker, 2012). Another example is a type of mutation that is frequently seen in cancer cells. In cancer cells, transverse type of RAS proto-oncogene is transformed into an oncogene by a mutation. With this transformation, the 12th codon GGC converts to GTC and causes the code to be read as valine (mis-sense mutation) instead of glycine during translation (Weinberg, 2014). The conversion of the serine amino acid to phenylalanine (in 310th codon), which also leads to hyperactivation of kinases in cancer cells, leads to disruption of protein-protein interaction and consequently disruption of the signal transduction pathway (Cocco et al., 2019). HGPRT (hypoxanthine-guanine phosphoribosyltransferase), which plays an important role in the metabolism of purines in patients with Lesch-Nyhan syndrome, deteriorates enzyme activity by mutational changes that may occur in the amino acids on the active sites of the enzyme (G69E, G70R, S103R, T167I, D193N, and D200G), so this deterioration leads to hypoxanthine accumulation (Miesfeld and McEvoy, 2017).

All of the point mutations may not alter the amino acid within the polypeptide sequence. Although this type of mutation changes the codon code, these mutations are called silent mutations because the amino acid in the polypeptide to be synthesized does not change (Cox et al., 2015).

Indel (Insertion or Deletion) Mutations

These are mutations caused by the introduction of new nucleotides into the ancestral DNA sequence or by the removal of nucleotides from the DNA sequence (Pierce, 2010; Cox et al., 2015). The deletion occurs as a result of the reverse repetitive sequences looping during replication and the DNA polymerase skips this loop structure, or as a result of the two strands separated in the regions where the repetitive sequences are separated and re-matched in a different position (with one or more base difference) (Srivastava, 2013). Deletion mutations are expressed as Δ (delta) (Snyder et al., 2013). For example, ΔF508, which is expressed for deletion in the CFTR gene, refers to the deletion of the codon encoding phenylalanine at the 508th position. Insertions are showed by the symbol "::" and indicated between the target gene and the inserting element (lacZ::Tn10 indicates that the Tn10 transposon is inserted into the *lacZ* gene (Clark, 2005). This type of microinsertions and microdeletions, which lead to very important changes, are caused by replication errors and larger indel mutations result from genetic recombination errors (Madigan et al., 2012). These genetic recombination errors are unequal crossovers between repetitive sequences localized on different DNA molecules or unequal recombinations between short repetitive sequences on the same DNA molecule (Srivastava, 2013). Indel mutations result in the reading frame being regenerated (causing normal ORF to change), causing in a sequence of triple codes (a new ORF) which results in the presence of completely different amino acids from the polypeptide sequence to be synthesized. All indel mutations do not cause frame shift (Pierce, 2010). In the case of changes in the input or output of nucleotides of 3 or in multiples of 3, to the polypeptide sequence that will be synthesized only one or more amino acids are introduced or one or more amino acids are removed from it (Table 1).

Indel mutations, which does not occur in multiples of 3 and 3, reach the dimensions that threaten the viability of the cell as it completely changes the amino acid sequence in the polypeptide chain to be synthesized. For this reason, indel mutations of living things in housekeeping genes (which cannot maintain cell viability without housekeeping genes) are not frequently implicated. Approximately 5% of spontaneous mutations in *E.*

coli consist of deletions (Clark, 2005). Indel mutations in haploid organisms, such as bacteria, are more harmful than diploid organisms. Indel mutations occurring in multiples of 3 and 3 may not be of a scale that threatens the viability of the eukaryotic cell. Because, there is another homologue that has not undergone indel mutation. However, if the same mutation occurs in the homologue, the living being is severely affected by this mutation. For example, living cells have a 250 kb (cystic fibrosis transmembrane conductance regulator) gene encoding a transmembrane protein that transfers the input and output of chloride ions to the cell. The 3 base pair deletions (ΔF508 deletion) of the CFTR gene, which encode phenylalanine at the 1514th, 1515th and 1516th positions result in a defective CFTR protein with an amino acid deficiency (Brown, 2012; Klug et al., 2015). This defective protein is also unable to adhere to the cell membrane and leads to a thicker mucus layer in the lungs. Various types of cancer develop as a result of the insertion of the DNA sequence leading to the formation of the amino acid sequence Tyr-Val-Met-Ala into the exon 20 region of the gene encoding HER2 protein (Paul et al., 2019). In the genome of familial hypercholesterolemia individuals, there are insertions in different regions along the LDLR (low density lipoprotein receptor) gene (Klug et al., 2015). While the ACCCC sequence is deleted at 150-155th positions, the TTCTGCAAACTCCTCCC sequence is inserted. As a result of this change, it is thought that the transcription to be reduced (De Castro-Oros et al., 2011). There are also insertions that are very important factors in ensuring the natural diversity of microorganisms (Dale and Park, 2010). Such insertions generally inactivate the gene. In the genome of an organism, the insertion or deletion of nucleotides of hundreds or even thousands of base pairs can lead to the complete loss of function of a gene or the acquisition of a new gene (Madigan et al., 2012). For example, in wild-type *E. coli*, a *bgl* cryptic gene begins to be expressed when a transposon promotor is inserted into the promotor of the *bgl* cryptic gene which is not expressed due to the defective promoter (Clark, 2005).

As a result of point mutations, there may be no amino acid changes in the polypeptide chain to be synthesized, or all amino acids in the polypeptide chain may change from one or more point mutation. With the formation or disappearance of stop codons as a result of mutation, the function of the functional polypeptide chain to be synthesized may be altered or may be completely destroyed. The formation of a new stop codon leads to premature termination of polypeptide chain synthesis during translation. The destruction of an existing stop codon also results in the expression of a longer polypeptide chain during translation. In both cases, the functionality of the protein to be synthesized may be affected.

Table 1. Point mutations

Point Mutation Type	Nucleotide Transformation
Transition	A→G or G→A (purine → other purine)
	C→T or T→C (Pyrimidine → other pyrimidine)
Transversion	C→G, T→A, C or T→G (pyrimidine → purine)
	A→C, A→T, G→C, or G→T (purine → pyrimidine)
Deletion	CAAGGAAGTT→ CAAGAAGTT Gln-Gly-Ser → Gln-Glu-Val
Insertion	CAAGGAAGTT→ CACAGGAAGTT Gln-Gly-Ser- → His-Arg-Lys-

Duplication

In a genome whose genomic integrity is preserved, when the number of copies of any DNA segment exceeds 2 is called duplication. Duplication has been discovered in Drosophila by the presence of flies with Barr's eye phenotype. In general, most genomes of eukaryotic organisms contain 2 copies of each DNA segment. In some cases, the number of available copies may be 3 and/or much more. For example, the 16A region, which should be a single copy on an X chromosome of a female *Drosophila melanogaster*, results in mutant Barr-eye flies that have 2 copies as a result of duplication. In individuals with Charcot–Marie–Tooth (peripheral nervous system disease leading to advanced atrophy of the distal limb muscles) in humans, a copy of the 17th chromosome has a duplicated region of 1.5 million bp

(Kumar and Eng, 2015; Jorde et al., 2016). The PMP22 gene, which encodes a component of peripheral myelin in this region, carries 2 copies due to duplication (Brown, 2012). Increased dosage of the product of the non-functional PMP22 duplicated gene contributes to demyelination. Interestingly, deletions in the same gene region result in a different hereditary neuropathic disease. The disease occurs in both cases where there is an increase or decrease in dosage of the PMP22 gene product (Jorde et al., 2016). However, it should be kept in mind that the presence of rRNA, immunoglobulin, olfactory receptor genes, which have a large number of copies in the genome where genetic integrity is preserved and do not cause a pathological condition. Duplications occur due to incorrect repair of chromosome fractures, unequal crossing-over, retrotransposition, and errors in DNA replication (Hartwell et al., 2011; Iñiguez and Hernández, 2017). Numerous duplications are also known to occur through mobile genetic elements. Numerous multiple gene copies and gene families occur in the genomes of eukaryotic organisms through mobile genetic elements (Craig et al., 2010; Hartwell et al., 2011; Nei, 2013; Krebs et al., 2018). This situation has an important place in genome evolution. Duplicated genes can be differentiated by neutral mutations in the evolutionary process to form new gene varieties/multiple gene families, or they can quickly be silenced and become pseudogenes (Krebs et al., 2018). For example, in the evolutionary process, the globin gene family has been able to produce pseudogenes belonging to globin genes and the formation of hemoglobin and myoglobin proteins through duplication and neutral mutations (Craig et al., 2010; Brown, 2012; Krebs et al., 2018). Another example is olfactory receptors responsible for smell, and is estimated to be about 1000 in the genome. This gene family is also derived by duplication from a common ancestral gene and subsequently differentiated by neutral mutations (Nussbaum et al., 2015).

Repeat Expansion

One of the classic examples that lead to genomic instability is the re-expansion due to problems encountered when replicating the unusual DNA template (Pavlov et al., 2006). There are three nucleotide specific DNA sequences that are repeated many times in the genomes of some living things (Klug et al., 2015). Due to the presence of these trinucleotide repeats in some regions of the DNA, the genome has unusual genetic instability (Allison, 2007). Increases in the number of trinucleotide copies are called expanding trinucleotide repeats (Cox et al., 2015). An increase in the number of repeats leads to the formation of abnormal secondary DNA structures such as intrastrand hairpins and triple- and quadruple-stranded DNA (Pavlov et al., 2006; Hanaoka and Sugasawa, 2016). DNA sequences with trinucleotide repeats in both protein-coding regions and non-protein-coding regions of the gene are hot spots for mutation formation (Brooker, 2012; Hanaoka and Sugasawa, 2016). An increase or decrease in the number of repetitive nucleotide copies occurs as a result of the formation of hairpin and/or other similar special structures of repeating regions during DNA replication, and a result of DNA polymerase skipping or replicating the same repetition without replication (Pierce, 2010; Krebs et al., 2018). In addition, transposable elements are known to play an active role in the formation of repeat sequences in high-structured eukaryotic organisms (Hanaoka and Sugasawa, 2016).

Repeat expansions causing more than 40 human diseases suhs as mental retardation, muscular atrophy, cranial dysplasia, and increased risk of prostate cancer (Pavlov et al., 2006). The number of CGG trinucleotides in the gene called FMR1 in the genome of a normal human is 60 and below. The number of repeats in individuals with fragile X syndrome can be hundreds or even thousands (Pierce, 2010; Turpenny and Ellard, 2017). It has been found that various genetic diseases occur as a result of increasing the number of copies of different replicated nucleotides (Allison, 2007; Pierce, 2010; Brooker, 2012; Watson et al., 2014; Cox et al., 2015; Griffiths, 2015). Furthermore, in contrast to the increase in trinucleotide repeats, DNA polymerase can continue to synthesize the hairpin structure prior to replication where these repeats occur, and after such hairpin structure, deletion occurs according to ancestral DNA (Brooker, 2012). Table 2 lists the diseases that appear depending on the number of replicated trinucleotides and tetranucleotides. CAG repeats encoding glutamine amino acids in the genomes of humans with Huntington's disease in the number 37-121 cause abnormal aggregation of the synthesized protein when translated and the disease develops (Klug et al., 2015).

Table 2. Sequence and number of repeat sequences in different genetic diseases[*]

Disease	Repeat Place	Repeat Sequence	Number of repetitive sequences in the genome of a normal individual	Number of repetitive sequences in the genome of a sick individual
Fragile X site A	5'-UTR	CGG	11-33	40-62
Fragile X site E	Promotor	CCG	6-25	> 200
Huntington Disease	Encoding sequence	CAG	9-37	37-121
Myotonic Dystrophy type 1	3'-UTR	CTG	5-37	50-4000
Myotonic Dystrophy type 2	Intron	CCTG	11-26	75- > 11000
Fragile site E	Promotor	CCG	6-25	> 200
Friedreich's Ataxia	Intron	GAA	17-22	200-900
Kennedy Disease	Encoding sequence	CAG	19-21	> 46
Oculopharyngeal muscular dystrophy (PABPN1)	Encoding sequence	GCG	6	8-13

[*] Allison, 2007; Pierce, 2010; Brooker, 2012; Cox et al., 2015; Griffiths, 2015; Jorde et al., 2016; Turpenny and Ellard, 2017.

Despite the negative characteristics of the presence of repeat sequences, it should be noted that some of them have important physiological functions by being involved in centromere and telomeres (Hanaoka and Sugasawa, 2016).

Frameshift Mutations

These are mutations that occur in the DNA sequence, altering the structure of the amino acids that an ORF will give. The frame shift mutation in the protein gene completely inactivates the protein to be synthesized by altering the amino acid sequence (Snyder et al., 2013). Such mutations occur as a result of insertion and deletion of nucleotides 1, 2 and 4 into the DNA sequence of the ORF. Nucleotide insertions or deletions of 3 and 6 do not lead to frame shift, only a lack or excess of 1-2 amino acids occurs in the polypeptide chain (Snyder et al., 2013; Klug et al., 2015). Such mutations are often found in regions with repetitive DNA sequences (Srivastava, 2013). Indel mutations in intron regions do not alter frameshift mutations because they do not alter the order of the polypeptide to be synthesized. In this respect, they are considered to be different from indel mutations. If one of the stop codons (UAG, UAA, UGA) is formed as a result of the frame shift mutation in the protein coding regions (exons), the reading of the code during translation may stop (Klug et al., 2015).

3.2. Causes of a Mutation

The mutation, defined as changes in a DNA sequence, can occur in different ways. These changes occur either as a result of normal cellular metabolism functions (intrinsic factors; spontaneous hydrolysis, replication errors, replicative stress, reaction with endogenous chemicals) or by environmental factors (extrinsic factors; UV, ionizing radiation, chemicals, viruses) (Tiwari and Wilson III, 2019). Mutations are divided into two groups as induced or spontaneous mutations according to the manner in which they occur. Mutations that occur as a result of cellular functions without the influence of external factors are called spontaneous mutations, while mutations created by mutagens under the influence of external factors are called induced mutations (Madigan et al., 2012). The rate of induced mutations among the total mutations in the genome of the organism is even less than 1% (Kondrashov, 2017). The distinctive feature of spontaneous mutations is that induced mutations are caused by environmental agents, while the causes of changes in DNA are caused by intracellular events (Brooker, 2012).

Spontaneous mutations and induced mutations can be explained in more details as follows.

3.2.1. Spontaneous Mutation

Spontaneous mutations occur as a result of DNA replication, DNA repair, and error(s) during recombination (Konrashov, 2017). Spontaneous mutations in the genome are the main source of all genetic variation (Van Straalen and Roelofs, 2012). Errors in DNA replication are often uncommon, with the exception of certain viruses, such as HIV, with a very high rate of spontaneous mutation (Brooker, 2012). However, among living things, the bacteria is the group that genetic variation can be observed in a short time. When *E. coli* cells cultured under normal laboratory conditions they multiply every 30 minutes, they reach maximum cell density (10^9 cells/ml) and 30 generations in approximately 10-15 hours (Dale and Park, 2010). At each cell division, approximately 3 nucleotides may change in 10^{10} nucleotides of each cell (Alberts et al., 2015). In a bacterial cell, due to the role of DNA pol I in the intermittent strand during replication, the error rate in the synthesized intermittent strand is greater than in the continuous strand in which DNA pol III (base selection and error recovery ability is higher than DNA pol I). Therefore, the rate of spontaneous mutation in the discontinuous strand is believed to be higher than that of the continuous strand (Temizkan, 2013). In eukaryotic organisms with very large genomes, this rate (mutation rate) is 10 times higher than bacteria (Madigan et al., 2012). In humans, different genes may be mutated at different rates (Hartwell et al., 2011). Thousands of lesions accumulate in the genomic DNA of a typical mammalian cell over a 24-hour period (Nelson and Cox, 2017). These changes are known to occur as a result of errors that occur during normal cellular functions. However, insufficient 3'-5' exonuclease activity that provides proofreading property of DNA polymerase and/or accumulated by-products in the cell due to hereditary metabolic defects may cause changes in DNA (Brown, 2012; Temizkan, 2013). Spontaneous mutations are best explained by the fluctuation test of Luria and Delbrück in 1943 with bacteria and T1 bacteriophage.

Although the genome of the organism is replicated with extremely high accuracy, during replication or DNA repair, error prone DNA polymerases can insert the wrong nucleotides into the synthesized new chain. Therefore, genomic changes occur in living organisms and these genomic changes contribute to genomic variants. Since natural damage in a gene is usually eliminated by natural selection, there are not many individuals with spontaneous mutations in natural populations (Temizkan, 2013). An example of spontaneous mutations in humans is the increased number of trinucleotide repeats. Before explaining the "Error-prone replication bypass" and "Errors introduced during DNA repair" mechanisms that lead to the formation of spontaneous mutations, it is important to briefly explain the function and properties of DNA polymerase in replication.

Functions and Properties of DNA Polymerases

DNA polymerases are enzymes that add dNMP (deoxynucleoside monophasphate) to the structure of DNA using dNTP (deoxynucleoside triphosphate) as substrate during DNA synthesis (Shanbhag et al., 2018). DNA polymerases involved in DNA synthesis are complex proteins that are able to distinguish between true and false nucleotides in the template DNA by their active domain at high efficiency (Watson et al., 2014; Kondrashov, 2017). Although all DNA polymerases have 3 different regions as palm, thumb, and fingers, they have different polymerization properties, catalytic activity, progressivity, and DNA template preference (McVey et al., 2016). In addition to replication of undamaged DNA, DNA polymerases are also required for replication and repair of damaged DNA (Pavlov et al., 2006). They are classified into 2 groups according to their function as replicative (required only during cell division to replicate the genome) and non-replicative (required during the cell cycle) (Shanbhag et al., 2018). DNA replication occurs in the 5'-3' direction by the DNA polymerase and performs one of the newly synthesized strands intermittently and the other continuously (Allison, 2007; Brown, 2012). The DNA polymerase performs a nucleophilic attack on both the 3'-OH group and the free dNTP as a result of the interaction of well-preserved Asp residues with Mg^{2+} ions (Gahlon et al., 2017; Nelson and Cox, 2017). This nucleophilic attack by DNA polymerase to the –OH group at the 3' end of the primer and to free dNTP gives the DNA polymerase the specificity to perform synthesis only in the 5'-3' direction (Snustad and Simmons, 2012; Watson et al., 2014). Because DNA polymerase only synthesizes in the 5'-3' direction, one of the strands is intermittently and the other is continuously synthesized (Pierce, 2012). The DNA polymerase enzyme has an active site that is used to catalyze the addition of dNTPs to the new strand to be synthesized against the template strand during replication, and owing to this active site, the DNA polymerase recognizes and adds nucleotides at extremely high efficiency (Watson et al., 2014). A total of 8 different (A, B, C, D, X, Y, RT, and AEP [archaeo-eukaryotic primase superfamily]) family of DNA polymerases identified so far. Five kinds them (DNA pol I, II, III, IV and V) found in prokaryotes, 15 varieties in eukaryotes (α, β, δ, ϵ, σ, γ, λ, μ, ϕ, η, κ, ι, ξ, θ and Rev1), and 3 varieties (Pol BI, Pol BII and Pol D) in archaea, and some of them serve as replicative enzymes, others are involved in repair or transcription synthesis (Allison, 2007; Pierce, 2012; Watson et al., 2014; Hanaoka and Sugasawa, 2016; Shanbhag et al., 2018). For example, in prokaryotes, DNA pol III is the main replicative enzyme, DNA pol I fills the gap after removing the RNA primers in the strand synthesized in the interrupted chain, DNA pol II takes a role in DNA repair mechanisms, DNA pol IV and V take an active role in the translesions synthesis (Allison, 2007). The 3'-5' exonuclease activity of DNA pol I and III allows the enzyme to correct errors (Voet et al., 2016; Nelson and Cox, 2017). DNA polymerases distinguish between dNTPs and ribonucleosides (rNTPs), which are approximately 30-200 times more common, by virtue of van der Waals interactions between amino acids in the active site of DNA polymerase (Watson et al., 2014; Tiwari and Wilson III, 2019). Thus, the differentiation of dNTPs with less concentration in the cell is distinguished from rNTPs. However, when replicating the human genome, approximately 1000 rNTPs can be added per replication by replicative DNA pol δ and ϵ (Kondrashov, 2017). If a change in the DNA polymerase activity leading to significant changes is not lethal for the cell, it can significantly affect the efficiency of replication leading to various human diseases (Pavlov et al., 2006). This is due to the change of amino acids in the active site region of the DNA polymerase. For example, the efficiency of replication of leucine to methionine at position 868, which leads to the disappearance of exonucleolytic proofreading activity in the active domain of DNA polymerase α and δ, is dramatically reduced, resulting in mutator phenotypes (Pavlov et al., 2006).

Table 3. Mammalian DNA polymerases and their functions

Polymerase	Family	3'-5' exonuclease activity	Process/Functions
α (alpha)	B	no	Primase, DNA replication, TLS, DSB repair, HR
β (beta)	X		BER, HR?
γ (gamma)	A	yes	mitochondrial replication and repair, HR, BER
δ (delta)	B	yes	DNA replication, TLS, DSB repair, HR, NER, BER
ε (epsilon)	B	yes	DNA replication, TLS, DSB repair, HR, NER, BER
ζ (zeta)	B	no	DNA replication, TLS, DSB repair, HR, somatic hypermutation
η (eta)	Y		TLS, somatic hypermutation, HR
θ (theta)	A	no	BER, TLS, ICL repair, NHEJ, somatic hypermutation, HR?
I (iota)	Y		TLS, BER? Specialized MMR?
κ (kappa)	Y		TLS, NER, HR
λ (lambda)	X		HR?, NHEJ, MMEJ/alt-EJ, V(D)J recombination, BER
μ (mu)	X		DSB repair: NHEJ, MMEJ/alt-EJ, V(D)J recombination
ν (nu)	A	No/A domain of *E.coli*	ICL repair, peptide adducts
Rev1	Y		TLS, scaffold protein
TdT	X		NHEJ, MMEJ/alt-EJ, V(D)J recombination
PrimPol			TLS, De novo synthesis of DNA, bypass of oxidative lesions

DSB: Double Strand Breaks; BER: Base Excision Repair, MMR: Mismatch Repair; NER: Nucleotide Excisinon Repair; HR: Homologous Recombination; TLS: Translesion Synthesis; ICL: Inter Cross-link; NHEJ: Non Homologous Exchange Joining; V(D)J: Variable-Diversity-Joining; altEJ: alternative end-joining

Spontaneous Mutation Mechanisms

Bases in cellular DNA are constantly damaged by spontaneous hydrolysis and oxidation events and other endogenous and environmental mutagens (Pavlov et al., 2006). The error rate of DNA in each replication cycle in *E. coli* is approximately one in 10 million and replicative DNA pol III performs polymerization of 750-1000 nucleotides per second (Clark, 2005; Temizkan, 2013). This low rate of error in DNA is ensured by the base selection of DNA polymerase, proofreading activity and DNA MMR (mismatch repair) mechanisms (Pavlov et al., 2006). Although DNA polymerase exits nucleotides that have accidentally entered the structure with its exonuclease activity, this activity is sometimes not fully achieved

(Klug et al., 2015). There is a possibility that 3 different nucleotides may accidentally enter the newly synthesized strands against each base in the template strand, and errors with mismatches if not corrected by the mismatch repair system they will remain as a permanent mutation in the DNA sequence as a result of the subsequent replication cycle (Watson et al., 2014). In both of the prokaryotes and eukaryotes due to the involvement of different polymerases in the intermittent strand error rate is about 20 times higher than continuous strand (Clark, 2005; Brown, 2006). In eukaryotes, the replisome (the enzyme-protein complex performing the replication), which adds approximately 100 nt per sec, may encounter 4 obstacles that may cause the replisome to stop and spontaneous mutations to occur: (1) the presence of DNA sequences containing short repeats, (2) coincidence with RNA polymerase (3) DNA polymerase inhibition by the DNA-protein complex, and (4) the presence of intolerable DNA damage (Kondrashov, 2017). If these obstacles are not eliminated, dynamic mutations occur (Pavlov et al., 2006). During the replication process, when the DNA polymerase encounters these obstacles, it either stops the synthesis or continues the synthesis by bypassing the parts of the obstacle (Kondrashov, 2017). Translesion (TLS) DNA polymerases are available to overcome difficulties that will lead to formation of dynamic mutations (Pavlov et al., 2006). Lesion skipping properties of such DNA polymerases is provided by the large and flexible active domain of the DNA polymerase and the use of non-canonical interactions in the process of base pairings (molecular matching between AT and GC pairs due to molecular shape compatibilty) (Boldinova et al., 2017; Gahlon et al., 2017). Spontaneous mutations occur due to misprocessing of the replication mechanism when performing replication of undamaged DNA, translesions polymerases that work with much less accuracy, which allow the damage to be tolerated during replication of damaged DNA, and failure to perform DNA damage repair (Kondrashov, 2017). Some DNA polymerases are able to synthesize very short DNA sequences, even though there are no template DNA. (Kondrashov, 2017). Insertion of such sequences into the genome results in insertional mutations.

In addition to the amino and keto forms of dNTPs that will enter the DNA structure, imino and enol forms, which are tautomers, limit the accuracy of DNA polymerase and cause it to enter DNA structure (Watson et al., 2014). When these alternative forms are introduced into the DNA structure, the correct insertion of the DNA polymerase by its 3'-5' exonuclease activity and its replacement is known as proofreading activity of DNA polymerase (Brooker, 2012; Nelson and Cox, 2017). Among eukaryotic replicative DNA polymerases, only DNA pol α has no exonuclease activity (Hanaoka and Sugasawa, 2016). Most errors in nucleotide selection of DNA polymerase are corrected by proofreading activity (Pierce, 2010). Proofreading activity decreases the error rate of DNA polymerase up to 10^{-7}. Thus, the occurrence of mutation is further reduced by proofreading activity, but mutation occurs when this activity and subsequent postreplication is not repaired (Watson et al., 2014). When DNA polymerase performing a synthesis, spontaneous mutation rates occur at high frequency if the proofreading ability, which enables the last inserted nucleotide to check the accuracy, is missing or damaged (Clark, 2005).

Error-Prone Replication Bypass

In order for DNA replication to take place in a healthy way, the DNA must be in an undamaged state. However, in some cases, there may be numerous lesions in the template DNA to be used for DNA synthesis, which prevents the replication fork from progressing. In such a case, the cell evolves to have DNA polymerases of different properties and functions that can overcome this condition. In the presence of a DNA lesion, there are specialized TLS DNA polymerases that allow replication to continue and can cause more mutations than progressive replicative enzymes (Hanaoka and Sugasawa, 2016). There are 11 TLS DNA polymerases of at least 5 families (A, B, X, Y, and AEP for archaeo-eukaryotic primase) related to different DNA damage response pathways (Quinet et al., 2018). In vertebrates, there are 5 types of TLS DNA polymerases, η, Rev1, ζ, κ and ι, which are members of the Y family, and the main role of these family members is replication of damaged DNA (Pavlov et al., 2006; Gao et al., 2017; Shanbhag et. al., 2018). While TLS DNA polymerases perform their functions, the newly synthesized strand cannot retain the original DNA template like replicative polymerases, and some mutations occur. Despite the need for normal growth and replication in yeasts, DNA polymerase ζ contributes to the production of more than half of the spontaneous mutations that occur (Pavlov et al., 2006). This is the proof of TLS DNA polymerases show mutagenic properties. Translesion synthesis is mutagenic for 2 reasons: (1) damaged bases are often miscoded (e.g., 8-oxoguanine can be deoxyadenosine matched), and (2) incorrectly enters the structure due to low corrective efficiency and low profreadnig activity (Sale, 2012). In the absence of DNA damage, replicative DNA polymerases show more stringent binding affinity to clamp protein PCNA (proliferating cell nuclear antigen) than TLS DNA polymerases, whereas TLS DNA polymerases bind to PCNA since replication stops in the presence of DNA damage (Hashimoto et al., 2017). When replicative DNA polymerases encounters a DNA lesion during replication, they bypass the site of the lesion, and after completing the task of TLS DNA polymerases, replicative DNA polymerases resume the synthesis process (Temizkan, 2013; Hashimoto et al., 2017). When replicative polymerases arrive at the site of the lesion, there is a temporary gap between the lesion and the onset of replication in the downstream direction of the lesion, which allows the DNA polymerase to make changes in the damaged area (Pavlov et al., 2006). After polymerase exchange, TLS DNA polymerases work in two stages: In the first stage, the REV1, Pol η, Pol ι, and Pol κ inserter polymerases insert a nucleotide against the DNA lesion that causes DNA replication to stop in the damaged area, and in the second stage an extender polymerase (Pol ζ) takes over the task instead of inserter polymerase and extends the synthesis by adding nucleotides along the lesion to the strand across the lesioned region (Hashimoto et al., 2017; Quinet et al., 2018). In human cells, in the absence of TLS pol ζ, pol η is mostly active on the intermittent strand and creates a mutational cost on this strand (Kreisel et al., 2019). Due to the larger catalytic domains of TLS DNA polymerases than replicative polymerases, both replication of non-complementary bases to the nucleotides in the template DNA strand during replication can be performed in the newly synthesized strand, as well as performing replication of the abasic sites and bulky adducts (Sale, 2012; Watson et al., 2014; Gao et al., 2017). The active domains of TLS polymerases, which are members of the Y family, are large enough to take dimers into structure at the same time (Pavlov et al., 2006). Since TLS DNA polymerases do not have 3'-5' exonuclease activities, they do not show proofreading activity to correct the error (Allison, 2007; Boldinova et al., 2017). Therefore, whether a true or a false nucleotide is inserted into the structure, it remains as the nucleotide. If errors are not eliminated by the DNA repair system, this will result in a permanent mutation in the genome. The error rate of TLS polymerases may differ from each other. For example, in the presence of Mg^{2+} ions as a cofactor of DNA polymerization, PrimPol replicates the undamaged DNA template and has an error rate of 10^2-10^5 nucleotides, often producing indel mutations (Boldinova et al., 2017). If there is a mutation in the gene encoding TLS DNA polymerases, the mutation frequency in the genome may be further increased. For example, in XP-V patients, a variant of Xeroderma pigmentosum disease, because the DNA pol η gene has been mutated, replication of the lesion site is performed by DNA pol and leading to a higher mutation rate (Gao et al., 2017; Kreisel et al., 2019).

Pol η has an important role in MMR (Mismatch repair) and in bypassing UV-induced cyclobutane primidine dimers in the presence of clustered lesions caused by oxidation (Garcia-Diaz and Bebenek, 2007; Quinet et al., 2018). Pol η is able to bypass 90% of the UV-induced primidine dimers (Pavlov et al., 2006). In addition, it was found that pol η is often required for bypassing the 8-oxoG lesion in the intermittent strand (Kreisel et al., 2019). Pol η also leads to somatic mutations that enable the diversity of immunoglobulin genes (Pavlov et al., 2006). Pol ι plays an effective role in bypassing UV photoproducts in mutated mutants of the pol η gene (McVey et al., 2016). In patients with XP-V, there is a tendency to mutate G:C ratio as a result of lack of pol η activity in somatic hypermutation (SHM) formation (Quinet et al., 2018). In addition, Pol η reduces the frequency of mutations induced by MMS (Methyl methanosulphonate) and can bypass N-2-acetylaminofluorene (AAF)-induced lesions (Pavlov et al., 2006).

Pol ι, unlike all known DNA polymerases, has a unique nucleotide placement feature (Pavlov et al., 2006). This DNA polymerase in mammals preferably places a G against a T (Chen and Furano, 2016). This may be useful in restoring genetic information in deaminated areas in C–G or C^{me}–

G pairs (Pavlov et al., 2006). Where there are consecutive Ts, it is only possible to place G against the first T, while A can be placed against the subsequent Ts (Pavlov et al., 2006).

PrimPol synthesizes TLS against UV-induced DNA damage and 8-oxoG lesions (Jain et al., 2018). PrimPol ("Prim" -primase, "Pol"-polymerase), which is able to re-start the paused replication fork, slows replication and induces replicative stress, resulting in the accumulation of DNA breaks and chromosome instability (even if DNA damage does not occur as a result of disruption of the enzyme) (Boldinova et al., 2017).

Pol ζ is responsible for bypassing UV-induced mutations with Rev1 (Garcia-Diaz and Bebenek, 2007). The loss of pol ζ in mammalian cells results in a dramatic increase in chromosome instability (Pavlov et al., 2006).

Pol Rev1 introduces a deoxycytosine against abasic domains, adducts, uracil, and templated guanines (McVey et al., 2016). Pol Rev1 places a C against G or against a non-coding lesion, such as the abasic domain in template DNA (Pavlov et al., 2006).

Pol ν is capable of bypassing major groove peptide adducts and residues of DNA crosslink repair (Shanbhag et al., 2018). Pol ν also has the ability to add a T against the G in the template (McVey et al., 2016).

In mammals, DNA polymerase preferably places nucleotide A against the AP regions and thymine glycols, and also bypasses the lesion by inserting nucleotides against the cyclobutane pyrimidine dimers or pyrimidine–6/4-pyrimidone photoproducts ([6,4] PP) (Pavlov et al., 2006; Shanbhag et al., 2018). Pol θ-inactivated mouse cells develop sensitivity to many mutagens such as MMS, γ-ray, UV-ray and cross-linking agents (Pavlov et al., 2006).

Pol λ and μ leads to frame shift mutations (Pavlov et al., 2006). Pol κ involved in the bypass of BPDE-induced polycyclic aromatic hydrocarbon (PAH) and DNA adducts and in the synthesis of DNA damaged by estrogen metabolites, and places C against the damaged G (Pavlov et al., 2006). In addition, there are important roles of Pol κ, Pol η, Pol ζ, Pol θ, PrimPol, and Rev1 TLS DNA polymerases in maintaining replication in regions where the B form of DNA is not present (such as G-quadruplexes) causing DNA replication to cease (Quinet et al., 2018). Pol ζ and Rev1 have been found to play a role in bypassing small hairpin structures that are very common in all genomes (Northam et al., 2014).

Overproduction of TLS DNA polymerases sometimes has a mutagenic effect. For example, overproduction of pol κ in mouse cells provides about 10-fold increase in spontaneous mutations, whereas overproduction of κ, η and ι polymerases in yeast cells does not have a mutagenic effect (Pavlov et al., 2006).

Bypassing the lesion or performing mutation-terminated transcription synthesis is a multiple process, and sometimes collaboration may be required which requires the participation of several DNA polymerases (Pavlov et al., 2006). From TLS DNA polymerases, human Rev1 polymerase cooperates with η, ι, and κ polymerases to replicate UV-damaged templates, whereas XP-V cells with pol η mutant co-operate with ζ, ι and κ polymerases to bypass cyclobutane primidine dimers (McVey et al., 2016). Approximately 100 amino acids at the C-terminus of Rev1 interact with polymerases ι, κ and η (Pavlov et al., 2006).

Errors Introduced during DNA Repair

Replication of human genomic DNA is carried out by α, δ and ε, while nucleotides that pol α have inadvertently introduced into the structure are removed from the structure by the 3'-5' exonuclease activity of pol δ (Shanbhag et al., 2018). Specialized TLS DNA polymerases, which perform replication of damaged DNA, can also play an active role in DNA repair (Quinet et al., 2018). Various repair mechanisms have been developed to remove nucleotides that have been inadvertently introduced into the DNA structure, either in the replication fork or after progression of the replication fork. While these repair mechanisms work, various TLS DNA polymerases are employed to fill gaps in the DNA. Translesion DNA polymerases, which are involved in repair mechanisms, are able to insert the wrong nucleotides while filling the gaps formed in the newly synthesized strand or DNA as a result of their activity (Kreisler et al., 2019). For example, pol κ plays a role in NER, pol ζ in ICL repair, pol η in HR, pol θ in BER, pol λ in BER and

NHEJ at the same time they insert the wrong nucleotides into the DNA structure (Garcia-Diaz and Bebenek, 2007).

In *E. coli* the DNA pol I, in eukaryotes pol δ, pol ε and pol κ are involved in NER (Nucleotide Excision Repair) repair mechanism (Garcia-Diaz and Bebenek, 2007). During NER, when synthesizing DNA, in the presence of low dNTP concentration, the replicative Pol δ and ε are replaced by pol κ (Quinet et al., 2018). Pol κ is also involved in bypassing the bulky adducts on DNA (Garcia-Diaz and Bebenek, 2007).

In the BER repair mechanism, AP regions are formed on DNA by removing damaged bases on DNA and these AP regions are repaired by BER (Base Excision Repair) repair system (Sierra and Gaivão, 2014; Klug et al., 2015). After the removal of AP domains, δ, ε, λ and θ polymerases play a role in addition to β polymerase, which plays a key role in filling the resulting gap (Pavlov et al., 2006; Garcia-Diaz and Bebenek, 2007). Pol θ is involved in bypassing lesions in AP areas and placing bases against 6-4 photoproducts (McVey et al., 2016). Replication of non-repairable AP domains is usually performed by Rev1 and η DNA polymerases, and as these sites are replicated, TLS DNA polymerases are susceptible to make errors, leading to the formation of SHM (Quinet et al., 2018). Approximately 50% of SHM mutations occur as a result of the catalytic activity of Rev1 while skipping AP domains, while the other 50% are caused by the error-prone activity of pol η while undamaged DNA is replicated (Quinet et al., 2018).

In the MMR repair mechanism, the gaps formed after the DNA glycosylases recognize and remove bases with false matches such as G-U and G-T are filled by polymerases involved in BER such as pol β (Garcia-Diaz and Bebenek, 2007).

In the interstrand crosslinks (ICLs) repair mechanism, the space in the single strand formed by removing part of the damaged strand is filled by pol ζ (McVey et al., 2016). In eukaryotic cells, pol ζ plays a key role in the repair of cross-links induced by agents such as psoralen, diepoxybutane and nitrogen mustard, as well as ν and θ polymerases are involved in ICL repair (Pavlov et al., 2006).

In addition, 3 of the replicative DNA polymerases are involved in homologous recombination (Pavlov et al., 2006). Of TLS DNA polymerases

Pol η and Pol ζ play a role in homologous replication, while Pol θ plays an important role in the HR and NHEJ events of DSB (Double Strand Breaks) repair (Quinet et al., 2018). In mammalian cells, some polymerases take their roles in the following mechanisms; Pol η in HR, Pol λ and μ in NHEJ, and Pol δ and ε in double-strand fractures (Garcia-Diaz and Bebenek, 2007). Polymerase λ is involved in filling short spaces of one nucleotide during DNA repair (Garcia-Diaz et al., 2009).

Depurination, deamination and tautomeric shifts resulting in chemical exchange of bases in nucleotides cause spontaneous mutations (Brooker, 2012).

Depurination

In a normal mammalian cell at 37°C during a 20-hour cell cycle period, approximately 10,000 purines are naturally lost in DNA, but the DNA repair system allows the repair of abasic areas (the region where the base is not present in the DNA) that are formed due to purine loss (Brown, 2012; Griffiths et al., 2015). Abasic areas are formed by breaking the unstable glycosidic bond between the deoxyribose sugar and the base. These abasic areas are highly cytotoxic for the cell (Snyder and Champness, 2007; Brooker, 2012; Voet et al., 2016; Miesfeld and McEvoy, 2017). DNA polymerase may not be able to insert a complementary base directly into the apurinic sites, and may insert a false non-complementary base, and ultimately lead to mutation (Srivastava, 2013). Normally, the abasic domains are recognized and repaired by the BER systems; however, where these abasic domains are not repaired during the successive replication cycle, the DNA polymerase will randomly place any of the 4 nucleotides against the abasic domain in the newly synthesized strand, and consequently spontaneous point mutations (Pierce, 2010; Brooker, 2012; Klug et al., 2015).

Deamination

The amino groups in the structure of nucleotides can be removed as a result of hydrolytic effects during cellular processes or chemical interactions of environmental agents (Allison, 2007). DNA may react with water to spontaneously induce apurinic/apyrimidinic (AP) site formation or demaination of cytosine by hydrolysis of the glycosidic bond (Tiwari and Wilson III, 2019). By deamination, the amino group (NH_2) in A and C is removed and converted from the amino form to the keto form, and A converted into hypoxanthine and C into uracil (Pierce, 2010; Klug et al., 2015; Krebs et al., 2018). C is the most mutated base in mammals (Chen and Furano, 2016). U (C→U) formed by deamination of cytosine in the pair G·C, if it cannot be corrected by repair systems, during the replication process U matches A to the pair A·T instead of the G·C pair in ancestral DNA; the hypoxanthine formed by the demination of A matches C to cause the A·T pair to eventually turn into a G·C pair (Brooker, 2012; Klug et al., 2015; Griffiths et al., 2015). If U is not recognized by the DNA repair enzyme uracil-DNA-glycosylase, which is formed by deamination of the C in the G·C pair and is still not paired with G, the G·C pair is permanently converted to the A·T pair (Srivastava, 2013). 5-methylcytosine is found in the genome of most eukaryotic species and matches G. Thymine resulting from the deamination of 5-methylcytosine matches A in a successive replication and causes the initial G·C pair to return to the A·T pair (G·C → G·5mC → G·T → A·T) (Brooker, 2012; Krebs et al., 2018). As a result of such a mutation, a normal base is introduced into the structure, which cannot be recognized by the repair mechanism and the mutation remains intact, so that CpG islets with methylated cytosines (about 1% of the human genome) in the genomes of eukaryotic organisms are hot spots for mutation (Pierce, 2010; Brooker, 2012; Srivastava, 2013; Klug et al., 2015; Chen and Furano, 2016; Krebs et al., 2018). Mutations may occur 10 times or even 100 times more than normal predicted mutation rates in hot spots (Krebs, et al., 2018).

During replication $G_{(keto)} \cdot C_{(amino)}$ and $A_{(amino)} \cdot T_{(keto)}$ Watson-Crick pairings do not cause any abnormalities, $T_{(enol)} \cdot G_{(keto)}$, $A_{(imino)} \cdot C_{(amino)}$, $A_{(imino)} \cdot G_{(keto)}$, $G_{(enol)} \cdot T_{(keto)}$, $A_{(amino)} \cdot C_{(imino)}$ matches result in mutations (Brown, 2012; Brooker, 2012).

Tautomeric Shifts
The keto forms of G and T as well as the amino forms of A and C, are stable and show normal Watson-Crick base pairing (Brooker, 2012; Watson

et al., 2014). As the keto and amino forms of the bases change to enol and imino forms as a result of chemical reactions, tautomeric bases with different coupling properties are formed (Brown, 2012; Srivastava, 2013). As an alternative to normal bases, transient changes in bases are called tautomeric shift (Brooker, 2012). More than 100 different oxidative modifications have been cataloged that cause tautomeric shifts for DNA (Voet et al., 2016). Although Watson and Crick have stated that tautomeric bases cause mutations for many years, Pierce (2010) found that there is no convincing evidence that tautomers cause mutations. The author stated that the DNA contains a small amount of tautomeric bases, and the mutation was caused by wobble interaction and/or protonated H, which was not suitable for Watson-Crick coupling principle (Pierce, 2010). Free radicals disrupt the stable forms of the bases, allowing them to match with different bases (Voet et al., 2016). Reactive oxygen species such as superoxide radicals $(O_2^{-)}$ hydrogen peroxide (H_2O_2), and hydroxyl radicals (OH), which are formed by-products of aerobic metabolism and processed by normal cellular processes, also change the chemical structure of the bases in DNA structure and ultimately lead to spontaneous lesions in DNA (Griffiths et al., 2015). The reason for the change in the stable coupling properties of the bases is that the protons shift from their initial position to another position on the same base (Pierce, 2010). One of the most common reactions of reactive oxygen species for DNA is the oxidation of guanine. One of several different forms of oxidized guanine product resulting from oxidative modification of base G is the most common and highly mutagenic 7,8-dihydro-8-oxoguanine (8-oxoG; containing an extra O atom relative to the guanine nucleotide (Voet et al., 2016; Ba and Boldogh, 2018). 8-oxoG matches A during DNA replication and allows the conversion of the base pair G · C to the base pair T · A (transversion) (Allison, 2007; Brooker, 2012; Voet et al., 2016). Thymidine glycols caused by oxidative damage cause DNA replication to stop if not repaired Griffiths, 2015). However, S-adenosyl-L-methionine (SAM), which acts as a reactive endogenous chemical and is required for the transfer of methyl groups, modifies it to O6-methylguanine that matches T in the replication process by adding a methyl group to guanine (resulting in a G→A transformation) (Tiwari and Wilson III, 2019).

Transposons

Another condition that causes spontaneous mutations is the movement of transposons in the genome of all organisms (Klug et al, 2015). Transposable elements have strong mutagenic properties and move within the genome (Srivastava, 2013). There are many different transposable elements, but this section will focus on the relationship between mutations and transposable elements. An enzyme, called transposase, provides the transposition movement of the transposon from one site of the host genome to another site, which can be replicative and conservative (Griffiths, 2015). This movement of the transposons within the genome may alter the ORF as a result of entering the protein-coding region, disrupting the function of the gene, leading to disruption of the transcription of the gene involved in regulator regions, causing chromosomal damage (double strand fracture, inversion, translocation, deletion, etc.) (Watson et al., 2014; Klug et al., 2015). Due to repetitive sequences at the ends of the transposable elements, when they show replicative transposition movement, an increase in the number of repetitive nucleotides occurs, this can lead to various diseases (Griffiths, 2015). More than half of the spontaneous mutations in *Drosophila* are due to the placement of transposable elements near a functional gene (Pierce, 2010). For example, certain diseases such as *white apricot* (w^a) mutation for eye color in *Drosophila* occur as a result of the insertion of transposons into the Drosophila genome (Griffiths, 2015). Wrinkled allele in peas (encountered by Mendel) is caused by the insertion of transposons into the pea genome (Snustad and Simmons, 2012). Although more than 45-50% of the human genome consists of transposons, most of these transposable elements in the human genome are inactive and have lost their transposition ability (Pierce, 2010; Watson et al., 2014). However, it is also known that diseases such as hemophilia A (factor VIII gene), hemophilia B (factor IX gene), neurofibromatosis (NF1 gene) and breast cancer (BRCA2 gene) are formed by insertion of at least 11 Alu sequences into human genes (Griffiths, 2015).

3.2.2. Induced Mutation

Earlier in this chapter, spontaneous mutations were defined as the changes in the genetic structure of the cell as a result of metabolism. Apart from its own metabolism (except for internal environmental conditions), the cell is also influenced by external factors. These environmental factors include mutagens known as DNA-damaging agents. Changes caused by mutagens in DNA are called induced mutations. We can examine the factors that cause induced mutations in 3 groups, as follows;

1. *Physical mutagens*: UV, Ionizing radiation
2. *Chemical mutagens*: Base analogs, deaminating agent, alkylating agents, intercalating agents
3. *Biological mutagens*: Viruses, transposons

The causes of induced genomic changes in eukaryotic organisms that may result in the development of various diseases. These are examined in more details in the following sections.

Physical mutagens

Physical mutagens include types of ionizing and non-ionizing rays such as UV rays, infrared (IR) rays, X-rays, γ -rays, α-particles, β-particles and fast moving neutrons.

In 1927, Hermann Müller found that X-rays caused mutations in Drosophila (Pierce, 2010). In the following years, the effects of physical mutagens on DNA have been investigated. The rays in the electromagnetic spectrum regions are radio waves, microwaves, infrared, visible light (750-380 nm wavelength), UV, X-rays, γ-rays and cosmic rays, respectively (Klug et al., 2015). The wavelength of the beam decreases and the energy increases as you move from radio waves to cosmic rays (Klug et al., 2015). Among these rays are X-rays currently used for imaging in medical diagnosis and these rays are mutagenic (Srivastava, 2013). DNA molecules are particularly sensitive to short wavelength and high energy physical agents (Brooker, 2012). X-rays (known as ionizers), gamma and cosmic rays produce free radicals that are chemically reactive molecules by deeply penetrating biological materials that are stable (Brooker, 2012; Klug et al., 2015). Depending on the type and intensity of ionizing radiation, mutations such as point mutation, insertion, deletion, or even mutation that stop DNA replication have a variety of mutagenic effects (Brown, 2012). Free radicals are chemical species containing one or more unpaired electrons, which can change the coupling properties of bases when interacting with electroactive DNA bases (Klug et al., 2015; Oliveira-Brett et al., 2019). For example, the interaction of guanine and adenine nucleotides with ROS (reactive oxygen species) produces 8-oxoG and 2,8-dyhydroxyadenine, and these products are highly mutagenic because A and G have lost their normal base-pairing specificity (Oliveire-Brett et al., 2019). Ionizing radiation, which has the property of removing electrons from atoms, damages the base structures in DNA and breaks the phosphodiester bonds (Pierce, 2010). However, although ionizing beams have a direct effect on DNA, they sometimes also ionize them by acting on other biomolecules, resulting in the formation of free radicals (Brown, 2012; Srivastava, 2013).

UV radiation at wavelength 200-300 nm (wavelength 254 nm is the most mutagenic) is between the 5th and 6th C atoms of thymine bases, often consecutive on the same DNA strand, and/or less often between the 4th C atom of cytosine and the 6th C atom of thymine creates a cyclobutyl ring and leads to the formation of primidine dimers or cross-linkage between two strands (Snyder and Champness, 2007; Srivastava, 2013; Griffiths et al., 2015; Voet et al., 2016). UV radiation penetrates only the surface of cells in plants and animals with high structure, does not lead to ionization (Snustad and Simmons, 2012). UV radiation, which has less energy than ionizing rays, disrupts the configuration of DNA with primidine dimers and prevents replication and possibly produces double strand breaks in DNA (Pierce, 2010; Miesfeld and McEvoy, 2017). UV-B causes direct lesion by forming cyclobutane primidine dimers, while UV-A causes indirect lesion by forming free radicals (Pecorino, 2012). Although the resulting primidine dimers are repaired immediately by the DNA repair system, sometimes the repair system may fail. It has already mentioned that Pol η and θ, among the TLS DNA polymerases involved in repair, bypass the lesioned site. In addition, UV radiation interacts with certain molecules in the cell (particularly riboflavin and tryptophan) including hydroxyl radicals and singlet oxygen to produce ROS (Miesfeld and McEvoy, 2017).

Another physical mutagen is heat. Heat stimulates the water-induced segment and breaks the β-N-glycosidic bond that binds the sugar in the nucleotide structure to the base and results in the formation of AP domains (Brown, 2012).

Chemical Mutagens

There are more than 80,000 hand-made chemicals of commercial importance and approximately 1000 new ones are added to these chemicals each year (Voet et al., 2016). It is almost impossible to avoid mutations in the genomes of organisms exposed to these chemicals, including mutagens that have serious effects (base analogues, deaminating chemicals, alkylating agents, intercalating agents, etc.). Some substances known to cause cancer by creating mutations in humans are: cigarette smoke containing nicotine, polycyclic aromatic hydrocarbons (PAH), benzo[a]pyrene (B[a]P), heterocyclic compounds (furan), N-nitrosamines, aldehydes (formaldehyde), volatile hydrocarbons (benzene), heavy metals, etc. Some of these substances (PAHs, benz[a]anthracene and B[a]P) are naturally generated from energy sources (such as coal, crude oil, and gasoline) in daily use and capable of inducing DNA damage directly or indirectly (Tiwari and Wilson III, 2019). Chemicals such as formaldehyde and acetaldehyde bind covalently to DNA, protein and other cellular nucleophiles and, if not repaired or hydrolyzed, they form DNA adducts, DNA-DNA cross-links, DNA-protein cross-links and/or DNA-glutathione adducts (Nohmi and Fukushima, 2016). Some chemicals are sufficiently similar to normal bases to enter the structure of the DNA. Such chemicals are called base analogs (Griffiths et al., 2015). DNA polymerase cannot distinguish between these base analogs and normal bases, so base analogs can enter the structure of the newly synthesized strand during DNA replication (Pierce, 2010). Once these chemicals have entered the structure of the DNA, they do not show the matching of the normal bases in the structure of the DNA. After replication, they cause the base analogue to match the base of the DNA that is not present in the ancestor DNA. As a result, base analogs cause mutations. For instance, the 2-AP (2-aminopurine) commonly used in research is an analogue of adenine base and can be matched to thymine (2-AP·T) as well as to the cytosine (2-AP·C) (Klug et al., 2015). If 2-AP gains protons, it can be matched with cytosine. As a result, in the original ancestral DNA the A·T pair is transformed into the G·C pair after 2-AP enters the DNA and replicates instead of Adenine (A·T → 2-AP·T→ 2-AP·C → G·C) (Srivastava, 2013; Griffiths et al., 2015). Alternatively, in the newly synthesized DNA strand, 2-AP is introduced into the cytosine by mismatch and then the 2-AP matches with thymine (C·G → C·2AP → T·2AP → T·A) (Pierce, 2010). Base analogs are commonly used as positive controls in mutagenicity/antimutagenicity tests such as the AMES test.

Another base analog is 5-BU (5-bromouracil), which is thymine analog. If this halogenated with Bromine from the 5th C atom of the pyrimidine ring performs a tautomeric shift to the enol form (Br in the structure increases this probability), 5-BU presents matching with guanine and as a result of replication after this pairing, the transforms from the T·A pair in the ancestor DNA into the C·G pair occurs (Klug et al., 2015). As there may be a conversion of a pair of T·A to a pair of C·G (T·A → 5-BU·A → 5-BU·G → C·G), there may be a vice versa (G·C → G·5-BU → A·5-BU → A·T) chance of a conversion (Pierce, 2010). 5-BU is sometimes used in cancer treatment because it enters the structure of DNA and causes numerous mutations and leads to cell death (Brooker, 2012). Unfortunately, 5-BU and similar chemicals used in cancer treatment do not only affect cancer cells but also normal cells. In addition to the possibility of such chemotherapeutics converting protooncogenes to oncogenes, they can also prevent undamaged tumor suppressor genes from functioning, disrupting the expression levels of genes acting on the cell cycle and ultimately leading to cancer in normal tissues.

Some chemicals may be covalently attached to bases. As a result of this bonding, the coupling properties of the bases change. Although deamination occurs spontaneously often, some chemicals interact with DNA to remove the amino groups in the DNA structure from the bases (Snyder and Champness, 2007). Such chemicals are *deaminating agents*. For example, HNO_2 (nitrous acid) causes the amino (=NH2) group in the bases to be replaced by the keto (=O) group (replacing the amino group in the cytosine and adenine with the keto group, respectively, resulting in uracil and hypoxanthine, respectively), and when the DNA is replicated modified bases do not match the appropriate bases in the newly synthesized strand (uracil matches adenine and hypoxanthine matches cytosine) (Brooker, 2012). Like HNO_2, which leads to the removal of the amino group in cytosine, hydroxylamine and bisulfite chemicals cause the G·C pair to turn into A·T pair or the A·T pair into the G·C pair (Snyder and Champness, 2007).

Chemicals such as nitrogen mustard, ethyl methanesulfonate (EMS), MMS, ethylnitrosourea, MNNG (N-methyl-N'-nitro-N-nitrosoguanidine) add alkyl groups (ethyl or methyl groups) to the bases or phosphate groups in the DNA (Pierce, 2010; Brooker, 2012; Snyder et al., 2013; Srivastava, 2013; Voet et al., 2016). Such chemicals are known as *alkylating agents*. Many reactive groups of bases are attacked by alkylating agents and the most reactive of these groups are the N7 positions of guanine and the N3 positions of adenine (Snyder et al., 2013; Cox et al., 2015). Alkylating agents often add an alkyl group to the positions of guanine O6 and N7, adenine N1, N3 and N7 and cytosine N1, leading to the formation of intrastrand or interstrand crosslinks that inhibit replication or transcription (Tiwari and Wilson III, 2019). The addition of the alkyl group by EMS or MMS from the N7 position of the guanine nucleotide and N3 position of the adenine nucleotide forms N7-methylguanine and N3-methyladenine, respectively (Srivastava, 2013). Alkylating agents such as nitrosoguanidine, which lead to significant deterioration in the structure of the helix, form O^6 methylguanine and O^4 methyl thymine, respectively, by adding the methyl group to the O^6 position of guanine and O^4 position of thymine (Snyder et al., 2013). It increases the susceptibility to hydrolysis of the glycosidic bond leading to loss of base with the occurrence of alkylation (Voet et al., 2016). Hydrolysis of the glycosidic bond results in the formation of an empty space in the DNA sequence (Tiwari and Willson III, 2019). The addition of alkyl groups to the DNA structure may not lead to a major deterioration in the structure of the helix, but may result in mutations while repairing lesions (Srivastava, 2013). Transversions occur as a result of primidine substitution of purine by error-prone enzymatic repair system (Voet et al., 2016). EMS, by adding an ethyl group to the structure of guanine O^6-ethylguanine showing thymin-forming properties. So, the transition of C·G pair to T·A pair occurs (Pierce, 2010).

Alkylating agents are extremely potent mutagens, and such agents are also used as chemotherapeutic agents in cancer treatment (cisplatin and cis-diamminedichloroplatinum) and in the treatment of malaria disease (acridine dyes) (Dale and Park, 2010; Snyder et al., 2013). Methylating agents (MNU and MMS) exhibit 20 times more reactive properties than ethylating agents (ENU and EMS), and repair of damage induced by ethylating agents is less efficient than repair of damage induced by methylating agents (Nohmi and Fukushima, 2016). It is estimated that alkylating agents, which generally cause transversions, spontaneously hydrolyze approximately 20,000 glycosidic bonds in each diploid human cell every day (Voet et al., 2016).

Intercalating agents are chemicals (proflavin, acridine orange, ethidium bromide, and dioxin) that create mutations by entering between adjacent bases in DNA (Pierce, 2010). Among these, Ethidium bromide, which forms the complex with DNA, is best known and used in molecular biology to determine DNA in experimental studies. Intercalating agents contain one or more cyclic rings and bind to purine or pyrimidine bases in DNA (Watson et al., 2014) Intercalating agents that exhibit their effect by direct inhibition of DNA replication are capable of settling at the center of the double helix between adjacent bases (Dale and Park, 2010; Brooker, 2012). Intercalating agents can shift between base pairs in the double helix, slightly unwind the helix, and thus increase the distance between adjacent base pairs (Brown, 2012). By interrupting or compressing the DNA bases, they disrupt the 3D helix structure of DNA and cause single nucleotide insertions and deletions that will cause frame shifts during replication (Pierce, 2010; Temizkan, 2013). Due to the structural breakdown of DNA by the intercalating agents, during replication the agents cause the DNA polymerase to either add one or more nucleotides against the intercalating agents or to skip one/more nucleotides due to the twist made by the intercalating agent (Watson et al., 2014). As a result, insertions or deletions of one or more bases occur (Snustad and Simmons, 2012). Intercalating agents can reverse the frame shift mutations they have created because they cause both single nucleotide insertion and single nucleotide deletion mutations (Pierce, 2012).

B[a]P, one of the most mutagenic chemicals distributed in the environment and foods, is metabolized by cytochrome P450 and epoxide hydrolase in the cell and produce (+)benzo[a]pyrene-7,8-dihydrodiol-9,10-epoxide (BPDE), which covalently binds to DNA. This adduct causes to transversion of G→T (Tiwari and Wilson III, 2019).

Biological Mutagens

Living things can be exposed to physical and chemical agents as well as biological agents. Viruses, transposons, plasmids, virions, which are biological agents, integrate their genomes into the host's genome when they enter the host organism. The function of the DNA sequence can also be altered by the integration of extra-host genetic information into the host's genome. The sequences of protooncogenes in the genome of eukaryotic organisms are similar to those in the genomes of viruses (Weinberg, 2014). This suggests that viral agents are involved in the eukaryotic genome in the evolutionary process. Although this process is seen spontaneously, we may consider them as inducing agents because of the high possibility of exposure to viruses such as influenza, which leads to epidemic diseases. Therefore, these can be evaluated in the category of inducing agents. In fact, promoters of various viruses are used in genetically modified organisms (GMOs) and these GMO products are offered for consumption as food. We do not have any clear information that strong promoters will not be included in our genome when we consume GMO products. The organisms that could not adapt to the changes in the host genome by biological agents were eliminated by natural selection, and the adaptive organisms evolved and survived. As previously described, transposons, the genome of a virus can alter or completely destroy its activity if integrated into a gene in the host's genome, transform the inactive pseudogenes into an active gene if integrated into a regulator sequence, disrupt the expression of the gene if integrated into a regulatory sequence, and if integrated into splice areas change the processing of RNA.

If the genome of retroviruses, possessing a strong promoter, is located in front of a proto-oncogen in the genome of the host cell, the proto-oncogen transforms into an oncogene, thereby causing the normal cell to become carcinogenic (Pierce, 2010). In addition, a strong promoter of the virus, in the case of its insertion in front of an enhancer sequence can change the expression of the gene (Allison, 2007). In addition, the virus may undergo mutation in such a way that it becomes a proto-oncogene oncogene during repeated infectious and proliferative cycles (Allison, 2007; Pierce, 2010).

In the 1970s, it was discovered that oncogenic viruses can induce gene mutations involving point mutation, insertion, and deletion in mammalian cells (Shapiro et al., 1984).

It has been found that after the injection of 9 non-infectious DNA and RNA-containing viruses for *Drosophila melanogaster* into males of this species, all of them are highly mutagenic, causing numerous gene mutations or microdeletions (Gershenson, 1986).

Cytomegalovirus, Rubella virus, Herpes virus, Human immonodeficieny virus (HIV), Human papilloma viruses (HPV) are examples of viruses that exhibit mutagenic effects in the organism (Salem, 2016; Prati et al., 2018). HIV-1 cause to high error rates due to the tendency of misincorporation and mismatch prolongation of reverse transcriptase (RT), which synthesizes error-prone DNA (because RT has no 3'-5' exonuclease activity) (Bakhanashvili et al., 2005). RT in the cytoplasm of HIV-1 infected cells efficiently places non-canonical dUTP into the structure of proviral DNA (Bakhanashvili et al., 2005; Saragani et al., 2018). Mutations occur as a result of both the misincorporation of dUTP and the integration of the virus genome into the host genome during repetitive replication cycles of the virus. Gene mutations caused by viruses in the host cell genome are most likely due to the introduction of viral DNA (or cDNA) fragments into the host cell genome (Gershenson, 1986).

Viruses have direct and indirect mutagenic effects on the genome. HPV oncoproteins act on different cellular pathways of the host cell and cause genomic alterations indirectly (Prati et al., 2018). For example, HPV E6 and E7 oncoproteins inhibit p53 and pRb, respectively. This allows replication of the DNA even in the presence of DNA lesions and results in the accumulation of DNA damage (Song et al., 1998). While E6 protein of different HPV types prevents the repair of UV-induced dimers in the host cell genome, studies showing that E7 inhibits X-ray repair cross-complementing protein 1 (XRCC1), which is effective in repairing fractures induced by ionizing radiation (Prati et al., 2018).

Inactivation of the DNA damage response (DDR) system, which plays an effective role in repairing DNA damage induced by oxidative stress or HPV proteins, results in inactivation of the cellular DNA damage response and accumulation of secondary mutations (Gupta and Mania-Pramanik, 2019).

4. EFFECTS OF GENE MUTATIONS

Mutations can either cause the DNA sequence to acquire a new function (such as the oncogene transformation of the proto-oncogene), or to cause loss of the function of the gene (such as inactivation of the p53 gene) or produce no functional change (Brown, 2012; Griffiths, 2015; Kumar and Eng, 2015). Such changes show varying degrees of effect from undetectable phenotypic to lethal effect on the organism. Mutations that increase the rate of mutation are called mutator mutations and such mutations occur in the DNA repair system-related genes or DNA polymerase genes (Pecorino, 2012). Mutations in the oncogene, tumor suppressor gene, or genes controlling the cell cycle, disrupt the proliferation of the cell, leading to the formation of clonal cell populations that is a typical characteristic of cancer cells (Basu, 2018). Approximately 100 types of human cancers are caused by mutations that result in the activation of protooncogenes or loss of activity of tumor suppressor genes (Bunz, 2016). These effects of mutations result in changes in the electroactivity of the protein/RNA that is the product of the gene sequence of interest, or disruption of the molecular interactions of other molecules that will interact with the protein/RNA (Oliveira-Brett et al., 2019).

If mutations occur in somatic cells, even though they are dominant, these mutations (***somatic mutations***) cannot be transferred to offspring individuals, they only manifest themselves in that somatic cell community (Temizkan, 2013). Although most somatic cell mutations lead to cell death, the loss of mutant cells is insignificant because there are many identical cells in the same tissue (Brown, 2006). However, the formation of mutant cell populations that will lead to tissue cancer (tumorization) is a threat to the organism. Nevertheless, such a situation is not passed on to the offspring. In order for the mutation to be transmitted to offspring individuals, it must occur in gamet cells or in cells that will give the gamet cells (*gametic mutations*) (Brown, 2012). If a child is born with a genetic disease that is not inherited from a parent, the mutations that cause this disease are called "*de novo mutations*". The majority of the observed cases of many autosomal dominant diseases are the result of de novo mutations (Jorde et al., 2016).

As a result of any mutation in a gene, a new allele of the gene is formed (Temizkan, 2013). Mutations that have little or no effect in the phenotype (silent mutations) lead to isoallel formation, while mutations that completely destroy the effect of the gene lead to the formation of a null allele (Snustad and Simmons, 2012; Temizkan, 2013). Mutations that inactive a gene are called *forward mutations*, and those that recycle these mutations are called *reversion mutations* (Krebs et al., 2018). Reversion mutation restores the original phenotype either by restoring the effect of the forward mutation to its original state or by suppressing it with a second mutation (Snustad and Simmons, 2012). If the mutation occurring in a second location suppresses the effect of a mutation, such mutations are called *suppressor mutations* (Snyder et al., 2013). For example, a mutation in the structure of the codon encoding an amino acid can be suppressed by a second mutation in the structure of the tRNA that will recognize that mutant codon, resulting in the correct amino acid entry into the polypeptide chain (Krebs et al., 2018). If suppressor mutations occur in the same gene, they are called *intragenic suppressor mutations*, and if they occur in a different gene, they are called *intergenic suppressor mutations* (Snyder et al., 2013). Suppressor mutations can restore nonsense, missense, and frameshift mutations to read them properly (Tamarin, 2001).

Most mutations are silent because they occur in the intergenic region (Brown, 2012). In prokaryotes that have very few non-coding regions in their genomes, the probability of silent mutations is much lower than in eukaryotes (Temizkan, 2013).

In the 5'-TTA-3' sequence encoding leucine, the 5'-TTA-3' sequence resulting from the A→G transition encodes the same amino acid. This type of mutation is called **synonymous mutation**. The 5'-AGA-3' sequence encodes arginine resulting from the transition of G→A in the 5'-GGA-3' sequence encoding glycine, a different amino acid, this type of mutation (which causes the coding of a different amino acid) is called as "**nonsynonymous mutation**" (Brown, 2012). Synonymous mutations are silent mutations because they do not change meaning even though they have changed the codon, and non-synonymous mutations are false meaning mutations because the meaning changes with codon change (Brown, 2006).

Mutations that cause decrease in a protein function or complete loss of function of the protein are called **LOF mutations** and mutations that lead to gaining a new function are called **GOF mutations** (Pierce, 2012). Most GOF mutations occur in regulatory sequences rather than coding regions (Brown, 2006). Mutations leading to functional gain sometimes result in the formation of a new protein product, more commonly it results in overexpression of the protein product or expression of it in the wrong tissues (Jorde et al., 2016; Brown, 2006). For example, the overexpression of the **bmeABC5** operon occurs as a result of the mutation of the GGTAAT sequence (G→T) of the GGGAAT IR (inverted repeat) sequence located in the IT1 region of the **bmeABC5** operon, which takes a place in the excretion of certain molecules in the membrane of **Bacillus fragilis** strains. This leads **B. fragilis** strains to gain resistance to antimicrobial drugs (Ghotaslou et al., 2018). While most of the mutations that cause loss of function show recessive features, mutations that gain function are dominant (Cox et al., 2015; Nussbaum et al., 2015). The reason for LOF mutations in diploid organisms being recessive is even one of the two copies of the gene's effect completely disappears, the second copy shows the effect (Brown, 2012). However, even if the organism is a dipoid, in some instances where the loss of function mutations are dominant, there are cases where the 50% loss of function mutation in one of the two copies cannot be tolerated, known as **haploinsufficiency** (Jorde et al., 2016). Haploinsufficiency is encountered in Marfan Syndrome that is caused by a mutation in protein gene of human fibrillin connective tissue (Brown, 2006). If the mutation prevents the organism from surviving when it causes loss of a gene product, such mutations are referred as *lethal mutations* (Temizkan, 2013). For example, a mutant bacterium that has lost the ability to synthesize an amino acid cannot grow and die in the absence of that amino acid (Klug et al., 2015). Because bacteria are haploid organisms, mutations in their genomes show their effects directly on the phenotype, so heredity is a strict rule (Temizkan, 2013). However, since eukaryotic organisms are diploid, recessive mutations show their effects on the phenotype only when they are homozygous (except for hemizygotism in their heterogametic state) (Snustad and Simmons, 2012). In other words, mutation in eukaryotes can create a phenotypic change depends on the dominant/recessive relationship. Even, it depends on the cell type and the time it occurs in the organism's life cycle (Temizkan, 2013). For example, mutations in the β globin gene, which have a dominant effect, begin to exert their clinical effects from the 2-6 months after birth (Jorde et al., 2016). In diploid organisms, mutations in the genes that are necessary for the growth of the organism are called *recessive lethal mutations* if they are homozygous for the offspring to cause death of the organism (Snustad and Simmons, 2012).

It is known that mutations contribute to natural diversity, but most of the mutations have deleterious effects, and are the source of many diseases and disorders such as cancer, hemoglobinopathies, hemophilia, Werner syndrome, Parkinson's disease, Huntington's disease, and Xeroderma pigmentosum (Nussbaum et al., 2015; Pierce, 2012; Klug et al., 2015). As previously stated, hereditary diseases may be caused not only by mutations in the exon regions, but also by mutations in the intron or regulatory regions. For example, there are specific sequences that allow the determination of the exon-intron boundary, which is very important in the splicing event, a step of processing pre-mRNA (Pierce, 2012; Allison, 2007). Mutations occurring in GT sequences recognizing the 5' splice domain (donor site) and/or AG sequences recognizing the 3' splice domain (acceptor site) are called *splice-site mutations* (Jorde et al., 2016). If the base change occurs in this specific sequence in the intron, the formation of a functional mRNA is prevented.

Such mutations in introns are deleterious mutations that can alter not only polypeptide production, but also the sequence of the polypeptide. Because the sequence regions to which the exon or intron will be truncated cannot be truncated due to the change and these sequences will enter the polypeptide sequence as amino acids. It is estimated that at least 15% of all genetic diseases in humans are caused by mutations affecting the splices (Berg et al., 2015). This suggests that mutations in introns should not be ignored when evaluating hereditary diseases.

Mutations in the mRNA resulting from the change in sequence of the stop codon to encode an amino acid as a result of mutation are called **readthrough mutation**. In such a case, it can tolerate short elongations without showing an effect on many protein functions, while longer elongations may inhibit protein folding and hence protein activity (Brown, 2012).

Whether the effect of a mutation is beneficial/harmful or with no effect, it is highly dependent on environmental conditions. The benefit of mutation is mostly at the population level. Non-lethal mutations leading to the formation of new alleles increase the occurrence of genetic variations in populations (Pierce, 2012; Klug et al., 2015). Without mutations, all genes would be of a single kind, alleles would not occur, and the organism would not have the ability to adapt to environmental changes. For example, the diversity of globin genes has occurred through mutations. ε and ζ globin genes are expressed in embryonic stage, γ and α globin genes in fetal stage and β and α genes in adult stage (Nussbaum et al., 2015). These different globin genes have also been formed through mutations in the evolutionary process. In addition to these changes that lead to the formation of normal hemoglobin molecules, it should be noted that there are changes that lead to the formation of abnormal hemoglobin molecules. Genetic damages related to human hemoglobin are the most common group of single-gene disorders. As a result of deletions occurring in three of the 4 α globin genes normally found in α thalassemia (while there is no clinical effect with deletion of one and/or two, severe α thalassemia as a result of deletion of three, and deletion of four cause lethality), severe β thalassemia develops as a result of nonsense, frameshift, and splice-site donor and acceptor mutations in the β globin gene (Jorde et al., 2016).

It is the FGF gene that encodes Fibroblast Growth Factor. The FGF gene contains only a few copies of the invertebrata genome, while the vertebrata genome contains more than 20 different FGF genes (Watson et al., 2014).

More than 10^8 varieties of antibodies that play an active role in the defense of the body against microbes occur through combinatorial association and somatic mutation (Berg et al., 2015).

In humans, the structure of the CCR5 protein changes (the CCR5Δ32 mutant is formed) with a deletion of approximately 32 amino acids (Δ32) that occurs on the surface of the helper T-cells and the CCR5 protein gene, a coreseptor protein for HIV-1. As a result of this change, the virus cannot recognize and enter the T-cell receptor (Cox et al., 2015; Klug, et al., 2015). Thus, although the individual carries HIV, the causative agent, does not develop AIDS.

Another useful example of mutation is the mutant HbS. Although HbS causes sickle cell anemia, if the individuals carrying this disease are heterozygous, they show resistance to malaria (Cox et al., 2015; Griffiths et al., 2015).

As a result of a single neutral mutation, since the function of the protein does not change, there is no situation that would affect reproduction or viability. These silent genetic alterations caused by neutral mutations are polymorphisms that cause different phenotypic features of organisms within the same species. However, it can be understood that neutral mutations that occur in other regions of the genome may have an effect on each other, so that neutral mutations may not actually be completely neutral.

5. CONCLUSION

All organisms living in the world are exposed to both spontaneous and induced mutations. We cannot avoid spontaneous mutations, but we can avoid the effect of mutations caused by inducing agents. This can be achieved by minimizing contact with inducing agents. But unfortunately, every year thousands of chemicals enter our lives, poisoning us and our environment. Therefore, it has become utopian for us to avoid inducing agents. Although repair mechanisms against mutations have been developed in the living cell, mutations escaping these repair mechanisms may be effective in living organisms. This effect of mutations can work for the benefit or harm of the organism, and may have no effect (neutral mutation). Neutral mutations can have an effect that can either contribute to or eliminate adaptation to the environment in the face of changing environmental conditions. Antibiotics used against microorganisms have caused the environment of microorganisms to change and microorganisms to develop adaptation against this change. The harmony they have developed is the result of mutation. For example, a mutation in the structure of the ribosomal protein S12 gene in *E. coli* made streptomycin to be ineffective on *E. coli* (Brown, 2006). The resistance to anticancer drugs used in cancer treatment is due to alterations in the genes of proteins/enzymes that play a role in metabolism related to the uptake and excretion of drugs, or changes in the expression levels of these genes (Swayden et al., 2018). Such a situation is probably due to alteration in the DNA sequences of protein/enzyme/RNA molecules that are effective on the expression of these protein/enzyme genes. A mutation in the genome of a cell can change the response of that cell to internal and external factors.

In general, the positive effect of the mutation does not occur at the organism level, but at the population level. It is rarely seen in individuals (such as the Δ32 mutation in the CCR5 gene). When researchers first discovered the mutation, they emphasized the harmful effects of the mutation. However, when it was understood that mutations did not only cause harm to the living things, they also tried to give an advantage to living things by making modifications in the genome of living things. Moreover, in recent years, CRISPR (Clustered Regularly Interspaced Short Palindromic Repeats) technology is used to reverse the mutation leading to diseases such as sickle cell anemia, Huntington's disease, cystic fibrosis, etc. Huang et al. (2015), Hoban et al. (2016), and Li et al. (2016) managed to reverse the mutation caused by sickle cell anemia *in vitro* using CRISPR/Cas9 technology. As it can be seen, identifying mutations that lead to genetic diseases is the main important point in the treatment of these diseases. In order to eliminate the abnormality caused by a mutation, it is necessary to know what the change in the genome is causing the mutation.

REFERENCES

Alberts, B., Johnson, A., Lewis, J., Morgan, D., Raff, M., Roberts, K. & Walter, P. (2015). *Molecular Biology of the Cell*. 6th Edition, Garland Science, Taylor & Francis Group, LLC, New York.

Allison, L. A. (2007). *Fundamental Molecular Biology*. First Printing. Blackwell Publishing, Australia.

Ba, X. & Boldogh, I. (2018). 8-Oxoguanine DNA glycosylase 1: Beyond repair of the oxidatively modified base lesions. *Redox Biology*, 14, 669-678.

Bakhanashvili, M., Novitsky, E., Levy, I. & Rahav, G. (2005). The fidelity of DNA synthesis by human immunodeficiency virus type 1 reverse transcriptase increases in the presence of polyamines. *FEBS Letters*, *579*, 1435–1440.

Basu, A. K. (2018). DNA Damage, Mutagenesis and Cancer. *International Journal of Molecular Sciences*, *19(*4), 970 doi:10.3390/ijms19040970, In Chemically-Induced DNA Damage, Mutagenesis, and Cancer: Basu, A. K. and Nohmi, T. MDPI, Basel, Switzerland.

Berg, J. M., Tymoczko, J. L., Gatto, G. J. & Stryer, L. (2015). *Biochemistry*. 8th edition, W. H. Freeman and Company, New York USA.

Boldinova, E. O., Wanrooij, P. H., Shilkin, E. S., Wanrooiji, S. & Makarova, A. V. (2017). *DNA Damage Tolerance by Eukaryotic DNA Polymerase and Primase PrimPol*. *18*, 1584, doi:10.3390/ ijms18071584. In Chemically-Induced DNA Damage, Mutagenesis, and Cancer: Basu, A. K. and Nohmi, T. MDPI, Basel, Switzerland.

Brooker, R. J. (2012). *Genetic Analysis Principles*. 4th edition, New York, The McGraw-Hill Companies, New York.

Brown, T. (2012). *Introduction to genetics, A Molecular Approach*, Garland Science, Taylor & Francis Group, LLC, New York and London.

Brown, T. A. (2006). *Genomes*, 3rd editidion. Garland Science, Taylor & Francis Group, LLC, New York and London.

Bunz, F. (2016). *Principles of Cancer Genetics*. Second edition, Springer Dordrecht Heidelberg New York-London.

Chen, J. & Furano, A. V. (2016). *Breaking bad: The mutagenic effect of DNA repair DNA Repair*, *32*, 43–51.

Clark, D. (2005). *Molecular Biology: Understanding the Genetic Revolution*. Elsevier Academic Press, China.

Cocco, E., Lopez, S., Santin, A. D. & Scaltriri, M. (2019). Prevalance and role of HER2 mutations in cancer. *Pharmacology & Therapeutics*, *199*, 188-196.

Cox, M. M., Doudna, J. A. & O'Donnell, M. (2015). *Molecular Biology, Principles and Practice*. Second Edition, W. H. Freeman and Company, New York.

Craig, N. L., Cohen-Fix, O., Green, R., Greider, C. W., Storz, G. & Wolberger, C. (2010). *Molecular Biology, Principles of Genome Function*. Oxford University Press Inc., New York.

Dale, J. W. & Park, S. F. (2010). *Molecular Genetics of Bacteria*. First imprinting, Wiley-Blackwell publishing, UK.

De Castro-Oro´s, I. Pampı´n, S., Bolado-Carrancio, A., De Cubas, A., Palacios, L., Plana, N., Puzo, J., Martorell, E., Stef, M., Masana, L., Civeira, F., Rodrı´guez-Rey, J. C. & Pocovi, M. (2011). Functional analysis of LDLR promotor and 5'-UTR mutations in subjects with clinical diagnosis of familial hypercholesterolemia. *Human Mutation*, Vol. 32, No. 8, 868–872.

Gahlon, H. L., Romano, L. J. & Rueda, D. (2017). Influence of DNA Lesions on Polymerase-Mediated DNA Replication at Single-Molecule Resolution. *Chemical Research in Toxicology*, *30*, 1972-1983.

Gao, Y., Mutter-Rottmayer, E., Zlatanou, A., Vazili, C. & Yang, Y. (2017). Mechanisms of post-replication DNA repair. *Genes*, *8(2)*, 64, doi:10.3390/genes8020064.

Garcia-Diaz, M. & Bebenek, K. (2007). Multiple functions of DNA polymerases. *CRC Crit Rev Plant Sci.*, *26*(2), 105–122.

Garcia-Diaz, M., Bebenek, K., Larrea, A. A., Havener, J. M., Perera, L., Krahn, J. M., Pedersen, L. C., Ramsden, D. A. & Kunkel, T. A. (2009). Scrunching during DNA repair synthesis. *Nature structural and molecular biology, 16*(9), 967-972.

Gershenson, S. M. (1986). Viruses as environmental mutagenic factors. *Mutation Research, 167*(3):203-213.

Ghotaslou, R., Yekani, M. & Memar, M. Y. (2018). The role of efflux pumps in Bacteroides fragilis resistance to antibiotics. *Microbiological Research, 210*, 1–5.

Gilbert, S. F. (2010). *Developmental Biology.* 9th Edition, Sinaucr Associates. Inc. Massachusetts, USA.

Gonzalez-Perez, A., Sabarinathan, R. & Lopez-Bigas, N. (2019). Local determinants of the mutational landscape of the human genome. *Cell, 177*, 101-114.

Greim, H. & Snyder, R. (2019). *Toxicology and Risk Assessment: A Comprehensive Introduction.* Second edition, John Wiley & Sons Ltd West Sussex, UK.

Griffiths, A. J. F., Wessler, S. R., Carroll, S. B. & Doebley, J. (2015). *Introduction to Genetic Analysis*, First Printing. W. H. Freeman and Company, USA.

Gupta, S. M. & Mania-Pramanik, J. (2019). Molecular mechanisms in progression of HPV-associated cervical carcinogenesis. *Journal of Biomedical Sciences*, 26-50. doi: 10.1186/s12929-019-0520-2.

Hanaoka, F. & Sugasawa, K. (2016). *DNA Replication, Recombination, and Repair: Molecular Mechanisms and Pathology.* Springer Tokyo Heidelberg New York Dordrecht London.

Hartwell, L. H., Hood, L., Goldberg, M. L., Reynolds, A. E. & Silver, L. M. (2011). *Genetics From Genes To Genomes.* 4th edition. The McGraw-Hill Companies Inc, New York.

Hashimoto, H., Hishiki, A. & Kikuchi, S. (2017). Structural basis for the molecular interactions in DNA damage tolerances. *Biophysics and Physicobiology, 14*, 199-205.

Hoban, M. D., Lumaquin, D., Kuo, C. Y., Romero, Z., Long, J., Ho, M., Young, C. S., Mojadidi, M., Fitz-Gibbon, S., Cooper, A. R., Lill, G. R.,

Urbinati, F., Campo-Fernandez, B., Bjurstrom, C. F., Pellegrini, M., Hollis, R. P. & Koohn, D. B. (2016). CRISPR/Cas9-mediated correction of the sickle mutation in human CD34+ cells. *Molecular Therapy, 24*(9), 1561-1569.

https://databeses.lovd.nl/shared/genes/DMD.

http://www.hgvs.org/content/databases-tools

https://omim.org/statistics/entry.

https://www.ncbi.nlm.nih.gov/clinvar.

https://www.ncbi.nlm.nih.gov/genome/?term=human+genome

https://www.omim.org/statistics/geneMap.

Huang. X., Wang, Y., Yan, W., Smith, C., Ye, Z., Wang, J., Gao, Y., Mendesohn, L. & Cheng, L. (2015). Production of gene-corrected adult beta globin protein in human erythrocytes differentiated from patient iPSCs after genome editing of the sickle point mutation. *Stem Cells, 33*(5), 1470-1479.

Iñiguez, L. P. & Hernández, G. (2017). The evolutionary relationship between alternative splicing and gene duplication. *Frontiers in Genetics*, doi: 10.3389/fgene.2017.00014.

Jain, R., Aggarwal, A. K. & Rechkoblit, O. (2018). Eukaryotic DNA polymerases. *Current opinion in Structural Biology., 53*, 77–87.

Jorde, L. B., Carey, J. B. & Bamshad, M. J. (2016). *Medical Genetics.* 5th edition, Elsevier Inc., Philadelphia.

Klug, W. S., Cummings, M. R., Spencer, C. A., Palladino, M. A. & Killian, D. (2015). *Concepts of Genetics.* 11th edition, Pearson Education, Inc., California, USA.

Kondrashov, A. S. (2017). *Crumbling Genome The Impact of Deleterious Mutations on Humans.* John Wiley & Sons, Inc., NJ, USA.

Krebs, J. E., Goldstein, E. S. & Kilpatrick, S. T. (2018). *Lewin's genes XII.* 11th edition. Jones & Bartlett Learning, LLC, Massachusetts, USA.

Kreisel, K., Engqvist, M. K. M., Kalm, J., Thompson, L. J., Boström, M., Navarrete, C., McDonald, J. P., Larsson, E., Woodgate, R. & Clausen, A. R. (2019). DNA polymerase η contributes to genome-wide lagging strand synthesis. *Nucleic Acids Research, 47*(5), 2425-2435.

Kumar, D. & Eng, C. (2015). *Genomic Medicine, Principles and Practice.* Second edition. Oxford University Press, New York.

Li, C., Ding, L., Sun, C. W., Wu, L. C., Zhour, D., Pawlik, K. M., Khodadadi-Jamayran, A., Westin, E., Goldman, F. D. & Townes, T. M. (2016). *Novel HDAd/EBV reprogramming vector and highly efficient Ad/CRISPR-Cas sickle cell disease gene correction.* Scientific Reports, 6:30422 DOI: 10.1038/srep30422.

Li, Y., Zhang, Y., Li, X., Yi, S. & Xu, J. (2019). Gain-of-function mutations: An emerging advantage for cancer biology. *Trends in Biochemical Sciences*, https://doi.org/10.1016/j.tibs.2019.03.009.

Madigan, M. T., Martinko, J. M., Stahl, D. A. & Clark, D. P. (2012). *Brock biology of microorganisms.* 13th edition. Pearson Education, Inc., Illinois, USA.

McVey, M., Khodaverdian, V. Y., Meyer, D., Cerqueira, P. G. & Heyer, W. D. (2016). Eukaryotic DNA Polymerases in Homologous Recombination. *Annul Reviews of Genetics*, *50*, 393–421.

Miesfeld, R. L. & McEvoy, M. M. (2017). *Biochemistry.* First edition, W. W. Norton & Company Ltd, Canada.

Nei, M. (2013). *Mutation-Driven Evalution.* First Edition. Oxford University Pres, UK.

Nelson, D. L. & Cox, M. M. (2017). *Lehninger Principles of Biochemistry.* 7th Edition, W. H. Freeman, New York, USA.

Nohmi, T. & Fukushima, S. (2016). *Thresholds of Genotoxic Carcinogens From Mechanisms to Regulation.* Elsevier Academic Press, Amsterdam, Boston, Heidelberg, London, New York, Oxford, Paris, San Diego, San Francisco, Singapore, Sydney, Tokyo.

Northam, M. R., Moore, E. A., Mertz, T. M., Binz, S. K., Stith, C. M., Stepchenkova, E. I., Wendt, K. L., Burgers, P. M. J. & Shcherbakova, P. V. (2014). DNA polymerases f and Rev1 mediate error-prone bypass of non-B DNA structures. *Nucleic Acids Research*, *42*(1), 290-306.

Nussbaum, R. L., McInnes, R. R. & Willard, H. F. (2015). *Thompson & Thompson Genetics in Medicine* 8th edition, Elsevier Inc., Philadelphia.

Oliveira-Brett, A. M., Diculescu, V. C., Enache, T. A., Fernandes, I. P. G., Chiorcea-Paquim, A. M. & Oliveira, S. C. B. (2019).

Bioelectrochemistry for sensing amino acids, peptides, proteins and DNA interactions. *Current Opinion in Electrochemistry*, *14*, 173-179.

Paul, P., Malakar, A. K. & Chakraborty, S. (2019). The significance of gene mutations across eight major cancer types, *Mutation Research-Reviews in Mutation Research*, *781*, 88-99.

Pavlov, Y. I., Shcherbakova, P. V. & Rogozin, I. B. (2006). Roles of DNA polymerases in replication, repair, and recombination in eukaryotes. *International Review of Cytology*, *255*, 41-132.

Pecorino, L. (2012). *Molecular Biology of Cancer: Mechanisms, Targets, and Therapeutics* Third Edition, Oxford University Press, Oxford.

Pierce, Benjamin A. (2010). *Genetics Essentials, Concepts and Connections*. First printing, W. H. Freeman and Company, New York.

Pierce, Benjamin A. (2012). *Genetics, Conceptual Approach*. 4th edition, W. H. Freeman and Company, New York.

Prati, B., Marangoni, B. & Boccardo, E. (2018). Human papillomavirus and genome instability: from productive infection to cancer. *Clinics*, doi: 10.6061/clinics/2018/e539s.

Quinet, A., Lerner, L. K., Martins, D. J. & Menck, C. F. M. (2018). Filling gaps in translesion DNA synthesis in human cells. Mutation Research, *Genetic Toxicology and Environmetantal Mutagenesis*, https://doi.org/ 10.1016/j.mrgentox.2018.02.004.

Sale, J. E. (2012). Competition, collaboration and coordination–determining how cells bypass DNA damage. *Journal of Cell Science*, *125* (7), 1633-1643.

Salem, M. S. Z. (2016). Pathogenetics. An introductory recview. *Egyptian Journal of Medical Human Genetics*, *17*(1), 1-23.

Saragani, Y., Hizi, A., Rahav, G., Zaouh, S. & Bakhanashvili, M. (2018). Cytoplasmic p53 contributes to the removal of uracils misincorporated by HIV-1 reverse transcriptase. *Biochemical and Biophysical Research Communications*, *497*(2), 804-810.

Schildgen, V. & Schildgen, O. (2018). The lonely driver or the orchestra of mutations? How next generation sequencing datasets contradict the concept of single driver check point mutations in solid tumours–NSCLC as a scholarly example. *Seminars in Cancer Biology*, https://doi.org/10.1016/j.semcancer.2018.11.005.

Shanbhag, V., Sachdev, S., Flores, J. A., Modak, M. J. & Singh, K. (2018). Family A and B DNA polymerases in cancer: Opportunities for therapeutic interventions, *Biology*, *7*, 5, doi:10.3390/biology7010005.

Shapiro, N. I., Marshak, M. I. & Varshaver, N. B. (1984). Mutagenic effects of DNA-containing oncogenic viruses and malignant transformation of mammalian cells. *Cancer Genet Cytogenet*, *13*(2), 167-79.

Sierra, L. M. & Gaivão, I. (2014). *Genotoxicity and DNA Repair A Practical Approach*. Springer New York Heidelberg Dordrecht London.

Snustad, D. P. & Simmons, M. S. (2012). *Principles of Genetics*. 6th edition, John Wiley&Sons, Inc., USA.

Snyder, L. & Champness, W. (2007). *Molecular genetics of bacteria*. 3th edition. American Society for Microbiology, Washington, USA.

Snyder, L., Peters, J. E., Henkin, T. M. & Champness, W. (2013). *Molecular genetics of bacteria*. 4th edition. American Society for Microbiology, Washington, USA.

Song, S., Gulliver, G. A. & Lambert, P. F. (1998). Human papillomavirus type 16 *E6* and *E7* oncogenes abrogate radiation-induced DNA damage responses *in vivo* through p53-dependent and p53-independent pathways. *PNAS*, *95* (5), 2290-2295.

Srivastava, S. (2013). *Genetics of Bacteria*. Springer New Delhi Heidelberg New York Dordrecht London.

Swayden, M., Iovanna, J. & Soubeyran, P. (2018). Pancreatic cancer chemoresistance is driven by tumor phenotype rather than tumor genotype. *Heliyon*, doi: 10.1016/j.heliyon.2018.e01055.

Tamarin, R. H. (2001). *Principles of genetics*, 7th edition. The McGraw-Hill Companies, USA.

Temizkan, G. (2013). *Molecular Genetics*. Second edition, Nobel Publishing, Istanbul.

Tiwari, V. & Wilson, III. D. M. (2019). DNA Damage and Associated DNA Repair Defects in Disease and Premature Aging. *The American Journal of Human Genetics*, *105*, 237–257.

Turpenny, P. D. & Ellard, S. (2017). *Emery's Elements of Medical Genetics*. 15th edition, Elsevier, China.

Van Straalen, N. M. & Roelofs, D. (2012). *An Introduction to Ecological Genomics*. Second Edition, Oxford University Press, New York, USA.

Voet, D., Voet, J. G. & Pratt, C. W. 0 (2016). *Fundamentals of Biochemistry Life At Molecular Level*. 5th edition, John Wiley & Sons, Inc., USA.

Watson, J. D., Baker, T. A., Bell, S. P., Gann, A., Levine, M. & Losick, R. (2014). *Molecular Biology of the Gene*. 7th Edition, Cold Spring Harbor, New York.

Weaver, R. F. (2011). *Molecular Biology*. 5th edition. The McGraw-Hill Companies, Inc., New York.

Weinberg, R. A. (2014). *The Biology of Cancer*. Second edition, Garland Science, Taylor & Francis Group, LLC, New York.

www.pathology.washington.edu/research/werner/databases/

In: Gene Mutations: Causes and Effects   ISBN: 978-1-53616-984-3
Editor: Helena M. Christoffersen   © 2020 Nova Science Publishers, Inc.

Chapter 2

GENE MUTATIONS OF HEREDITARY MOTOR NEURON DISEASES

Haruo Shimazaki, MD, PhD*

Division of Neurology, Department of Internal Medicine,
Jichi Medical University School of Medicine, Tochigi, Japan

ABSTRACT

Hereditary motor neuron diseases can be grouped into three categories. Those with upper motor neuron involvement are called hereditary spastic paraplegias (HSP), those with lower motor neuron involvement are referred to as spinal muscular atrophy (SMA), distal hereditary motor neuropathy (dHMN), Charcot-Marie-Tooth disease (CMT), and those with combined upper and lower motor neuron involvement are designated as familial amyotrophic lateral sclerosis (FALS). They are caused by mutations in the various genes. Recent advances in next-generation sequencing have discovered new causative genes or those mutations. We could identify several gene mutations in HSP, CMT, and FALS families using whole-exome or genome sequencing. In this review, we described the phenotypes and gene mutations and

---

* Corresponding Author's Email: hshimaza@jichi.ac.jp.

discussed genotype-phenotype correlations compared with previous reports.

1. HEREDITARY SPASTIC PARAPLEGIAS

Hereditary spastic paraplegias (HSPs) comprise a heterogeneous group of neurodegenerative diseases characterized by gradually progressive spasticity and weakness of the lower limbs with the predominant feature of a length-dependent degeneration of upper motor neurons. HSPs are classified by their mapped genetic loci, SPG1–SPG80. To date, about 70 causative genes have been identified, transmitted by autosomal-dominant, autosomal-recessive (AR), X-linked recessive inheritances, with *de novo* mutations also described. Clinical and genetic heterogeneity led us to use next-generation sequencing (NGS) technologies to genetic diagnosis for HSPs [1]. The most common HSP is SPG4, This is inherited as an autosomal dominant trait, and is associated with mutations in the *SPAST* gene [2].

1.1. SPG4

Table 1. Autosomal dominant spastic paraplegia families with *SPAST* mutations

Family No.	1	2	3	4	5
onset (proband)	47	15	45	45	30
age at examination	70	30	50	48	74
cognitive impairment	-	-	-	-	-
leg spasticity	+	+	+	+	+
other features	constipation	psychosis	-	-	ichthyosis
SPAST variants (NM_014946.3)	c.1137-8insA	c.1454 C>T	c.1245+1G>A	c.1504A>T	c.1210-1212 delTTT
AA consequences	p.L380fs	p.A485V	exon 9 skipping	p.K502*	p.F404del

SPG4 is the most frequent HSP characterized by pure spastic paraplegia, sometimes associated with dementia [3]. Intrafamilial variation of the symptoms or onset age was known widely.

We previously reported two autosomal dominant pure spastic paraplegia families [4, 5]. They had *SPAST* gene mutations. We encountered an additional three families with *SPAST* mutations (Table 1).

1.1.1. Family 1

The pedigree of the family is presented in Figure 1. The affected patients had spasticity, exaggerated tendon reflexes in the lower limbs and a Babinski sign. Blood samples were obtained with informed consent from affected and unaffected individuals. The proband suffered from severe constipation and occasionally led to paralytic ileus. Genomic DNA was extracted from peripheral blood leukocytes. We performed linkage analysis in the family and observed a probable linkage to chromosome 2p previously (data not shown).

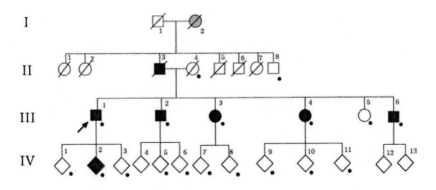

Figure 1. The pedigree of family 1.

This family includes eight affected persons (generations I, II, III and IV), and shows an autosomal dominant mode of transmission. In generation IV, gender concealed in those individuals denoted by a diamond shape to maintain the anonymity of the family (Modified from [4]).

SPAST NM_014946.3: c.1137-8insA, p.Leu380fs

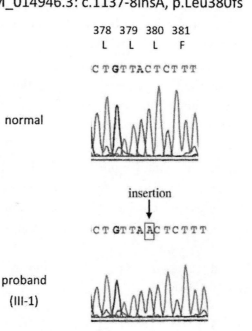

Figure 2. The sequence analyses of the proband (III-1) and normal family member.

The patient had a single nucleotide insertion mutation (c.1137-8 insA) in exon 8 of the *SPAST* gene (Modified from [4]).

Then, two affected members and two aged normal individuals in the present family were screened for mutations in the *SPAST* gene. According to the conditions reported previously [6], the 17 coding exons of the *SPAST* gene were amplified by polymerase chain reaction (PCR) from genomic DNA and sequenced directly. Concerning exon 8, an amplified fragment was subcloned into plasmids. Clones were then analyzed by restriction endonuclease digestion and sequencing. When sequence analysis revealed an insertion mutation (NM_014946.3: c.1137-8 ins A) (Figure 2) in exon 8 in the patient, its co-segregation with the disease was confirmed in the analyses of the other family members. This insertion variant will result in a frameshift with a premature stop.

1.1.2. Family 2

The family tree shows in Figure 3. The patients had spasticity, exaggerated tendon reflexes in the lower limbs and Babinski signs. The proband and his brother (IV-11) sometimes developed psychosis. Blood samples were obtained from the three patients and 12 individuals at risk in the family with informed consent. Linkage analysis showed a probable linkage to chromosome 2p (data not shown). One patient and one aged normal individual in the present family were screened for variations in the *SPAST* gene.

As the sequence analysis revealed a missense mutation (NM_014946.3:c.1454C>T, p.A485V) (Figure 4) in exon 12 in the patient, its cosegregation with the disease was then ascertained in the rest of the family.

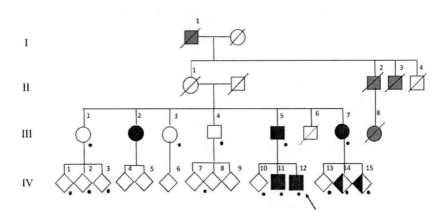

Figure 3. The pedigree of family 2.

The pedigree includes nine affected persons (generations I–IV), four symptomatic carriers and an asymptomatic carrier (generation IV) in four generations, and exhibits an autosomal dominant mode of transmission. In generation IV, the gender is concealed for those individuals denoted by diamonds to maintain the anonymity of the family (Modified from [5]).

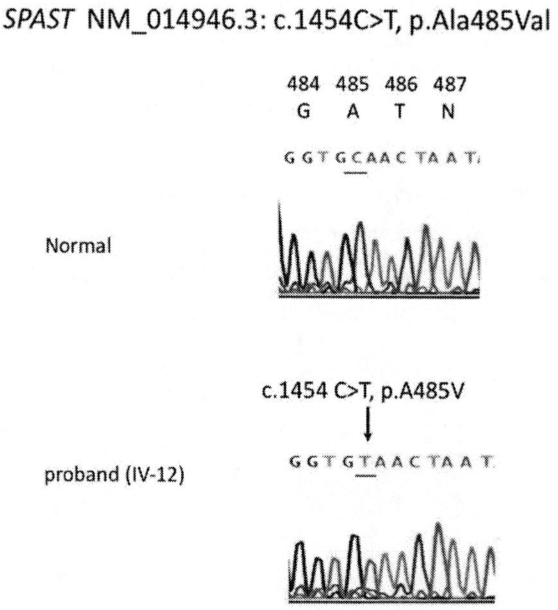

SPAST NM_014946.3: c.1454C>T, p.Ala485Val

Figure 4. The sequence analyses of the proband (IV-12) and normal family member.

The patient had a missense variant (NM_014946.3:c.1454C>T, p.A485V) in exon 12 of the *SPAST* gene (Modified from [5]).

1.1.3. Family 3

This family included three patients over the three generations (Figure 5). The mother (I-2, Figure 5) and son (III-1, Figure 5) of the proband (II-1, Figure 5) had spasticity, exaggerated tendon reflexes in the lower limbs and a Babinski sign. The proband noticed gait disturbance in the age of 45. He visited our clinic at age 50. Neurological examination revealed pure spastic paraplegia.

Blood samples were obtained from the proband and son with informed consent. Whole-exome sequencing and subsequent sanger sequencing disclosed a splicing variant (NM_014946.3: c.1245G>A) in intron 9 of the *SPAST* gene (Figure 6). This variant was previously reported as an aberrant splicing mutation and result in skipping of exon 9 demonstrated by cDNA sequencing [7]. The proband suffered from his right equinovarus foot deformity. We treated with botulinus toxin A injection into his right leg muscles.

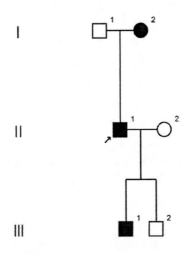

Figure 5. The pedigree of family 3.

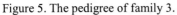

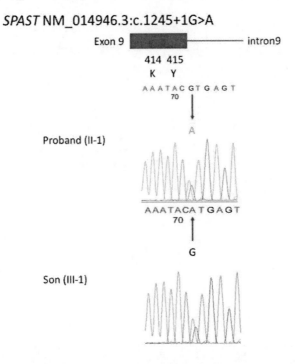

Figure 6. The sequence analyses of the proband (II-1) and affected son (III-1).

The patients had a splicing variant (NM_014946.3:c.1245G>A) in intron 9 of the *SPAST* gene.

1.1.4. Family 4

This family included two patients over the two generations (Figure 7). The proband and her mother had spasticity, exaggerated tendon reflexes in the lower limbs and a Babinski sign. The proband (II-2, Figure 7) noticed gait disturbance in the age of 45. He visited our clinic at age 48. Neurological examination revealed pure spastic paraplegia. Her mother (I-2, Figure 7) suffered from spastic paraplegia since the age of 60.

Blood samples were obtained from the proband and her mother with informed consent. Whole-exome sequencing of the proband's DNA and subsequent Sanger sequencing identified a novel nonsense variant (NM_014946.3: c.1504 A>T) in exon 13 of the *SPAST* gene (Figure 8). This variant led to a stop codon at amino acid residue 502. This nonsense variant was not registered in public databases, considered a novel mutation.

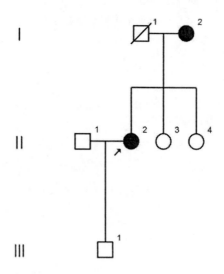

Figure 7. The pedigree of family 4.

Proband and her mother suffered from spastic paraplegia. Proband is ambulatory, whereas her mother is wheelchair-bound.

SPAST NM_014946.3: c.1504A>T, p.Lys502*

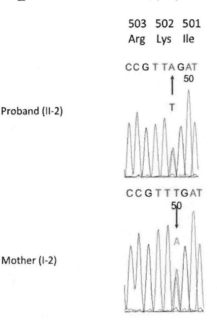

Figure 8. Mutation analysis of family 4.

Sanger sequencing (the reverse direction) of the proband and her mother DNAs identified a novel nonsense variant (NM_014946.3: c.1504 A>T) in exon 13 of the *SPAST* gene.

1.1.5. Family 5

A 74-year-old woman visited our clinic because of her gradually worsening gait disturbance since the age of 30. She suffered from ichthyosis in her legs. Neurological examination revealed bilateral leg spasticity, exaggerated tendon reflexes in the lower limbs and a Babinski sign. Her father had also shown gait disturbance while he was alive (Figure 9).

Blood samples were obtained from the proband with informed consent. Whole-exome sequencing of the proband's DNA and subsequent Sanger sequencing identified a three-base deletion (NM_014946.3: c.1210-1212 del TTT, p.F404del) in exon 9 of the *SPAST* gene (Figure 10). This deletion was a pathogenic variant of the *SPAST* gene reported previously (8). No mutations were identified in the *ALDH3A2* gene, a responsive gene for Sjögren-Larsson syndrome.

Haruo Shimazaki

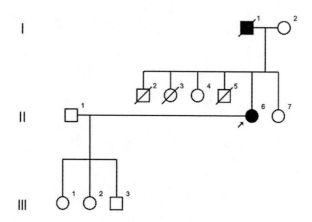

Figure 9. Family pedigree of the family 5.

SPAST NM_014946.3:c.1210-1212delTTT, p.F404del

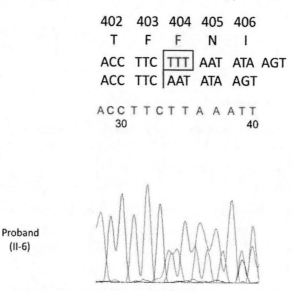

Figure 10. The sequence analyses of the proband (II-6).

The patients had a three-base deletion (NM_014946.3: c.1210-1212delTTT) in exon 9 of the *SPAST* gene.

1.2. SPG2

Spastic paraplegia type 2 (SPG2) is characterized by spastic paraplegia, autonomic dysfunction, normal intelligence, and normal lifespan. The responsive gene is proteolipid protein 1 (*PLP1*) gene, which is also caused in Pelizaeus-Merzbacher disease, displaying neonatal stridor, nystagmus, seizures, severe hypotonia followed by spastic quadriparesis, severe cognitive impairment and death before 10 years of age [9].

The proband (III-2, Figure 11) was pointed out his delayed psychomotor development at the age of ten months. He was diagnosed as cerebral palsy. His spastic paraparesis gradually worsened, so he became wheelchair-bound at age 18. He has no family history. Brain MRI disclosed white matter hyperintensity on T2-weighted images. He was referred to our clinic at age 31. The neurological examination revealed gaze-evoked nystagmus, spastic paraplegia, exaggerated DTRs of his legs and positive Babinski signs. His Mini-Mental State Examination (MMSE) was 26/30.

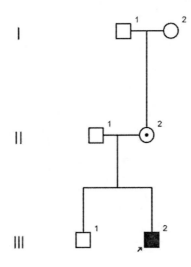

Figure 11. SPG2 family.

The proband (III-2) showed early-onset spastic paraplegia. His grandmother was demented, mother suffered from depression and brother showed mental impairment.

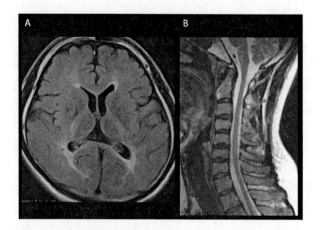

Figure 12. Brain and spinal MRI of the proband.

Brain FLAIR MRI (A) showed white matter abnormal intensities in internal capsules and occipital lobes. Cervical spinal cord T2-weighted MRI (B) showed no abnormal findings.

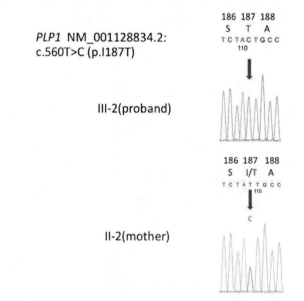

Figure 13. Sequence analyses of the proband and his mother's DNA.

A hemizygous *PLP1* mutation (NM_001128834.2: c.560T>C) was revealed on the X-chromosome of the proband (III-2). The same heterozygous *PLP1* mutation (NM_001128834.2: c.560T>C) was identified in his mother (II-2).

FLAIR images of brain MRI (Figure 12 A) showed white matter abnormal intensities in internal capsules and occipital lobes.

DNA analyses were performed for the patient and his mother with informed consents. We performed whole-exome sequencing in the proband. We confirmed the mutation by Sanger sequencing.

Whole-exome sequencing identified a hemizygous *PLP1* mutation (NM_001128834.2: c.560T>C) in the patient (Figure 13). A heterozygous *PLP1* mutation (NM_001128834.2: c.560T>C) was identified in his mother. This *PLP1* variant was already reported and called a rumpshaker mutation [10]. This mutation led to spastic paraparesis, congenital nystagmus and increased signal on cerebral T2-weighted MRI [11]. These clinical findings are consistent with those of the patient.

1.3. SPG17

SPG17 is called Silver syndrome, is an autosomal dominantly inherited disease characterized by spasticity of the legs and amyotrophy of the small hand muscles. SPG17 has usually the heterozygous missense variants in the gene Berardinelli-Seip congenital lipodystrophy type 2 (*BSCL2, seipin*) [12]. Biallelic null mutations in the *BSCL2* gene result in autosomal recessive Berardinelli-Seip congenital lipodystrophy type 2 [13].

The proband (II-1, Figure 15) was indicated his abnormal gait at the age of 18 and noticed intrinsic hand muscle atrophy at the age of 34. At age 52, he noticed frequent muscle cramps and atrophy of his lower legs. He visited our clinic at age 54. His father (I-I, Figure 15) suffered from gait disturbance and his son (III-1, Figure 15) noticed leg muscle cramps. Neurological examination revealed distal muscle weakness and wasting of the upper and lower limbs (Figure 14). All deep tendon reflexes were exaggerated except for the Achilles tendon reflex. His walking showed steppage and spastic gait. Nerve conduction studies revealed axonal neuropathy. His son showed only leg muscle cramps and exaggerated DTRs. His father did not allow us to his neurological examination and genetic test.

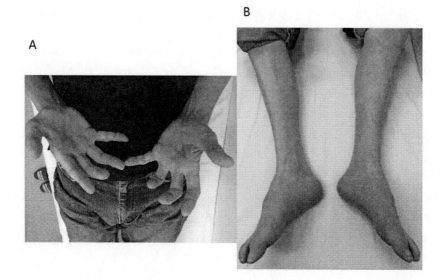

Figure 14. Hand and foot photography of the proband (II-1).

Intrinsic hand muscle atrophy (A), distal muscle atrophy of the leg and pes cavus foot deformity were noted (B).

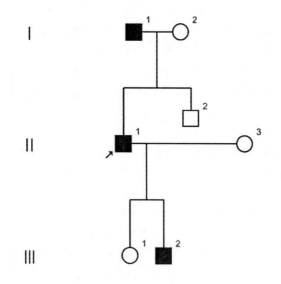

Figure 15. Family tree of the SPG17 family.

BSCL2 NM_032667.6: c.263A>G, p.Asn88Ser

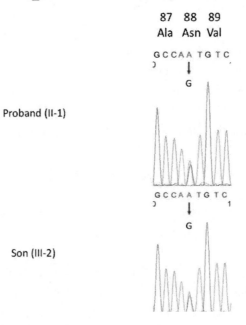

Figure 16. Sequence analysis of the proband (II-1) and his son (III-2).

A heterozygous *BSCL2* gene mutation (NM_035667.6: c.263A>G) was identified in the proband (II-1) and son (III-2).

DNA analyses were performed for the patient and his son with informed consents. We performed whole-exome sequencing in the proband. We confirmed the mutation by Sanger sequencing.

Whole-exome sequencing identified a heterozygous *BSCL2* mutation (NM_035667.6: c.263A>G) in the patient (Figure 16). The same heterozygous *BSCL2* mutation (NM_035667.6: c.263A>G) was identified in his son (Figure 16). This *BSCL2* variant was already reported from Caucasian [12] and Japanese [14]. Spastic paraplegia and distal muscle atrophy were consistent with symptoms of previously reported patients, although prominent muscle cramps were a characteristic feature of our cases.

1.4. SPG11

SPG11 is the most common type of autosomal recessive (AR) HSP. SPG11 shows early-onset spastic paraplegia with thin corpus callosum, mental impairment, and neuropathy [15, 16]. A sagittal image of Brain MRI shows thin corpus callosum (TCC). HSP with thin corpus callosum (TCC) is a feature associated with SPG1, SPG11, SPG15, SPG18, SPG21, SPG44-47, SPG49, SPG54, SPG56, SPG63, SPG67, SPG71, and so forth.

Spatacsin, the causative gene for SPG11, was identified (16). SPG11 cases usually had biallelic null mutations in the *Spatacsin* gene.

A non-consanguineous family including one patient. The proband (II-2) shows spastic paraplegia with TCC. Other members are all healthy. The father (I-1), the mother (I-2) and sibling (II-1) were neurologically asymptomatic.

The patient (II-2, Figure 17) noticed his gait difficulty at age 13. His gait disturbance was gradually worsened and wheel-chair bound at age 23. He had a mental impairment (MMSE 17/30). His brain MRI showed marked thin corpus callosum. (Figure 18) He treated with intrathecal baclofen administration at age 31 because of severe spasticity and pain of his legs.

We performed whole-exome sequencing (WES) of the patient's DNA and searched deleterious mutations of HSP genes in the WES result. Mutations were confirmed by Sanger sequencing and co-segregation study in this family. To evaluate the missense variant in exon 14 affected splicing, we extracted mRNA from the patient's leukocytes. RT-PCR was performed to investigate the effect of the variant on splicing, designing primers on exon 14 and 15.

Whole-exome sequencing (WES) could identify a novel nonsense mutation in exon 6 and a missense mutation in exon 14 of the *SPG11* gene, which is the causative gene for SPG11. The compound heterozygous mutations were confirmed by Sanger sequencing, co-segregated within this family (Figure 19).

The symptoms of this patient were identical to those of SPG11. We identified the novel nonsense mutation (p.Q389*) of the *SPG11* gene. We also identified missense mutation (p.I870V)[17], resulting in aberrant splicing [18].

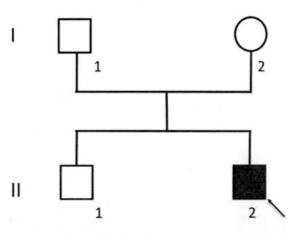

Figure 17. Family tree with an SPG11 patient.

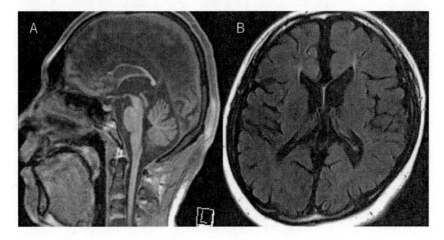

Figure 18. Brain MRI findings of the patient (II-2)

Sagittal T1 image showing a thin corpus callosum, especially the anterior part. Axial FLAIR image showed subtle ears of the lynx formation at the anterior periventricular portions of the lateral ventricles.

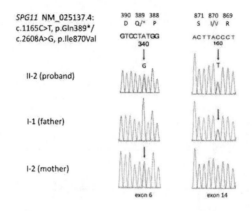

Figure 19. Result of sequence analysis.

Sanger sequencing (reverse sequences) confirmed the nonsense mutation
(NM_025137.3:c.1165C>T, p.Q389*) and missense one (NM_025137.3: c.2608A>G,
p.I870V) of the *SPG11* gene in the proband (II-2). This mutation was co-segregated with
the disease in this family.

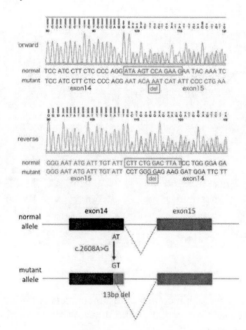

Figure 20. RT-PCR analysis of the proband's mRNA

Forward and reverse sequence analysis of RT-PCR product showed that c.2608A>G
substitution generated a new splice donor site (AT>GT), resulting to delete 13bp of exon
14.

2. CHARCOT-MARIE-TOOTH DISEASES

Charcot-Marie-Tooth diseases (CMTs) are a group of inherited neuropathies characterized by distal weakness, sensory loss, reduced or absent deep tendon reflexes and foot deformities. CMTs are a heterogeneous group of disorders clinically or genetically [19]. The causative genes for CMTs have been identified over 100 genes, we applied next-generation sequencing technologies to diagnostic approaches for CMTs [20].

2.1. CMT4D

Charcot-Marie-Tooth disease type 4D (CMT4D) is a demyelinating form of CMT characterized by a severe distal motor and sensory neuropathy with deafness, inherited an autosomal recessive manner in the Gypsy community. N-Myc downstream-regulated gene 1 (*NDRG1*) is a responsible gene for CMT4D [21].

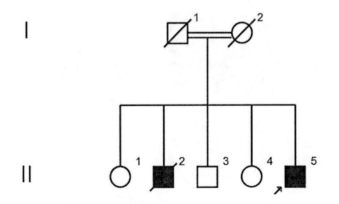

Figure 21. CMT4D family tree. Proband (II-5) and his deceased brother (II-2) with consanguineous parents showed the same phenotypes.

The proband (II-5, Figure 21) sometimes tended to fall in his elementary school periods. He could run slowly until his junior high school. He underwent foot surgery due to clubfoot deformities at the age of 16. He was diagnosed as 'muscular dystrophy'. At age 62, he and his brother (II-3) visit our clinic.

His father and mother were first cousins with each other. His deceased brother showed gait disturbance at the age of 2. He also underwent foot surgery due to clubfoot deformities at the age of 17. He noticed his hearing impairment at the age of 28. He used a wheelchair from the age of 40. He died from pneumonia at the age of 55.

Neurological examination of the proband revealed severe distal muscle wasting and weakness (Figure 22). He could stand and walk with assistance. Deep tendon reflexes were all absent, glove and stocking type sensory disturbance was noted. He suffered from severe deafness. Nerve conduction studies in his extremities could not evoke action potentials because of his severe neuropathy. His brain MRI was unremarkable.

DNA analyses were performed for the proband (II-5) and his brother (II-3) with informed consents. We performed whole-exome sequencing in the proband. We confirmed the mutation by sanger sequencing.

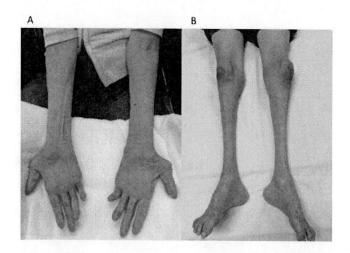

Figure 22. Severe distal hand (A) and leg (B) muscle atrophy of the proband (II-5).

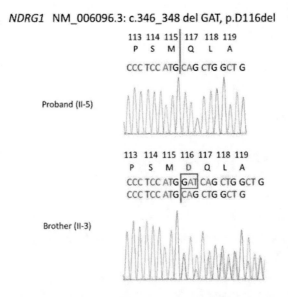

Figure 23. Sanger sequencing analysis of proband (II-5) and asymptomatic brother (II-3). A homozygous *NDRG1* three-base deletion (NM_006096.3: c.346_348 del GAT) in the proband (II-5) was identified. The same heterozygous *NDRG1* mutation (NM_006096.3: c.346_348 del GAT) was identified in his brother (II-3).

Whole-exome sequencing identified a homozygous *NDRG1* three-base deletion (NM_006096.3: c.346_348 del GAT) in the proband (Figure 22). The same heterozygous *NDRG1* mutation (NM_006096.3: c.346_348 del GAT) was identified in his brother (Figure 23). This *NDRG1* variant was a novel one and not registered in public databases. We consider the variant would be a pathogenic mutation.

3. AMYOTROPHIC LATERAL SCLEROSIS

Amyotrophic lateral sclerosis (ALS) is a fatal neurodegenerative disorder characterized by progressive weakness and atrophy of extremities, bulbar paresis, and respiratory failure. Most of ALS cases are sporadic, about 5-10% of ALS cases have a family history [22]. Until now, many causative genes for familial ALS (FALS) were identified. In Asians, most frequent FALS have superoxide dismutase 1 (*SOD1*) gene mutations, while in Europeans, most common FALS gene mutations are hexanucleotide repeat expansions in the *C9orf72* gene and *SOD1* is a second most frequent one [23].

3.1 ALS1(SOD1)

SOD1 was discovered as the first gene in 1993 associated with FALS (ALS1), which was inherited as an autosomal dominant trait (24). ALS1 patients with *SOD1* mutations presented slower progression and longer duration of disease, earlier age of onset, compared to those with sporadic ALS [25]. Over 100 mutations in the *SOD1* mutations were reported previously [26].

The proband (II-1, Figure 24) noticed his right foot weakness and gait disturbance at the age of 71. Three years later, he became aware of right-hand grip weakness. He referred to our hospital at the age of 74. His brother (II-3, Figure 24) was diagnosed ALS at the age of 60 in the other hospital. On neurological examination of the proband, right side and leg dominant muscle weakness and atrophy in his extremities, diminished or absent DTRs were noted. We could not detect his upper motor neuron signs. Nerve conduction study revealed marked decreasing of compound muscle action potentials. Needle EMG disclosed active neurogenic pattern.

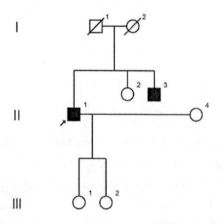

Figure 24. Family tree of the ALS1 family.

DNA analyses were performed for the proband (II-1) with informed consents. We performed whole-genome sequencing in the proband. We confirmed the mutation by Sanger sequencing.

Whole-genome sequencing identified a heterozygous *SOD1* mutation (NM_000454.4: c.380 T>C) in the proband (Figure 25). This *SOD1* variant was considered as a novel mutation. The nonsense mutation was located in the same amino acid position (NM_000454.4: c.380 T>A) was previously reported [27]. We consider this variant (c.380T>C) would be a pathogenic mutation.

We tried to riluzole administration and subsequent edaravone infusion therapy. But his weakness was gradually progressed and wheelchair-bound at the age of 77.

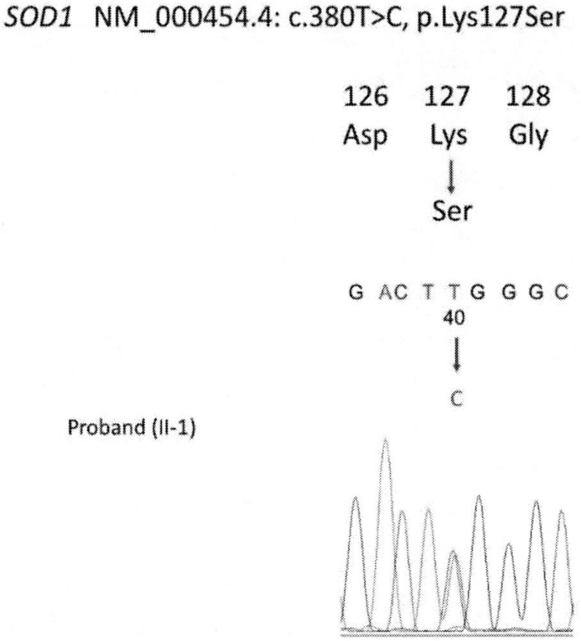

Figure 25. Sequence analysis of the proband. The novel *SOD1* gene variant (NM_000454.4: c.380T>C) was identified.

ACKNOWLEDGMENTS

We thank Japan Spastic Paraplegia research Consotium (JASPAC) for the *SPAST* gene analysis (SPG4 Family 3, II-1). We also thank Prof. Sonoo, Department of Neurology, Teikyo University School of Medicine for electrophysiological studies of SPG17 patient (II-1, Figure 15), and Dr. Ogino, Department of Neurology, Kitasato University School of Medicine for the information of FALS (SOD1) patient. (II-3, Figure 24).

REFERENCES

[1] Parodi L, Coarelli G, Stevanin G, Brice A, Durr A. Hereditary ataxias and paraparesias: clinical and genetic update. *Curr Opin Neurol.* 2018;31(4):462-71.

[2] Shribman S, Reid E, Crosby AH, Houlden H, Warner TT. Hereditary spastic paraplegia: from diagnosis to emerging therapeutic approaches. *Lancet Neurol.* 2019.

[3] White KD, Ince PG, Lusher M, Lindsey J, Cookson M, Bashir R, et al. Clinical and pathologic findings in hereditary spastic paraparesis with spastin mutation. *Neurology.* 2000;55(1):89-94.

[4] Namekawa M, Takiyama Y, Sakoe K, Shimazaki H, Amaike M, Niijima K, et al. A large Japanese SPG4 family with a novel insertion mutation of the SPG4 gene: a clinical and genetic study. *J Neurol Sci.* 2001;185(1):63-8.

[5] Namekawa M, Takiyama Y, Sakoe K, Nagaki H, Shimazaki H, Yoshimura M, et al. A Japanese SPG4 family with a novel missense mutation of the SPG4 gene: intrafamilial variability in age at onset and clinical severity. *Acta Neurol Scand.* 2002;106(6):387-91.

[6] Hazan J, Fonknechten N, Mavel D, Paternotte C, Samson D, Artiguenave F, et al. Spastin, a new AAA protein, is altered in the most frequent form of autosomal dominant spastic paraplegia. *Nat Genet.* 1999;23(3):296-303.

[7]   Svenson IK, Ashley-Koch AE, Gaskell PC, Riney TJ, Cumming WJ, Kingston HM, et al. Identification and expression analysis of spastin gene mutations in hereditary spastic paraplegia. *Am J Hum Genet.* 2001;68(5):1077-85.

[8]   Park SY, Ki CS, Kim HJ, Kim JW, Sung DH, Kim BJ, et al. Mutation analysis of SPG4 and SPG3A genes and its implication in molecular diagnosis of Korean patients with hereditary spastic paraplegia. *Arch Neurol.* 2005;62(7):1118-21.

[9]   Cailloux F, Gauthier-Barichard F, Mimault C, Isabelle V, Courtois V, Giraud G, et al. Genotype-phenotype correlation in inherited brain myelination defects due to proteolipid protein gene mutations. Clinical European Network on Brain Dysmyelinating Disease. *Eur J Hum Genet.* 2000;8(11):837-45.

[10]   Kobayashi H, Hoffman EP, Marks HG. The rumpshaker mutation in spastic paraplegia. *Nat Genet.* 1994;7(3):351-2.

[11]   Naidu S, Dlouhy SR, Geraghty MT, Hodes ME. A male child with the rumpshaker mutation, X-linked spastic paraplegia/Pelizaeus-Merzbacher disease and lysinuria. *J Inherit Metab Dis.* 1997;20(6):811-6.

[12]   Windpassinger C, Auer-Grumbach M, Irobi J, Patel H, Petek E, Horl G, et al. Heterozygous missense mutations in BSCL2 are associated with distal hereditary motor neuropathy and Silver syndrome. *Nat Genet.* 2004;36(3):271-6.

[13]   Magre J, Delepine M, Khallouf E, Gedde-Dahl T, Jr., Van Maldergem L, Sobel E, et al. Identification of the gene altered in Berardinelli-Seip congenital lipodystrophy on chromosome 11q13. *Nat Genet.* 2001;28(4):365-70.

[14]   Minami K, Takahashi S, Nihei Y, Oki K, Suzuki S, Ito D, et al. The First Report of a Japanese Case of Seipinopathy with a BSCL2 N88S Mutation. *Intern Med.* 2018;57(4):613-5.

[15]   Shibasaki Y, Tanaka H, Iwabuchi K, Kawasaki S, Kondo H, Uekawa K, et al. Linkage of autosomal recessive hereditary spastic paraplegia with mental impairment and thin corpus callosum to chromosome 15q13-15. *Ann Neurol.* 2000;48(1):108-12.

[16] Stevanin G, Santorelli FM, Azzedine H, Coutinho P, Chomilier J, Denora PS, et al. Mutations in SPG11, encoding spatacsin, are a major cause of spastic paraplegia with thin corpus callosum. *Nat Genet.* 2007;39(3):366-72.

[17] Crimella C, Arnoldi A, Crippa F, Mostacciuolo ML, Boaretto F, Sironi M, et al. Point mutations and a large intragenic deletion in SPG11 in complicated spastic paraplegia without thin corpus callosum. *J Med Genet.* 2009;46(5):345-51.

[18] Pippucci T, Panza E, Pompilii E, Donadio V, Borreca A, Babalini C, et al. Autosomal recessive hereditary spastic paraplegia with thin corpus callosum: a novel mutation in the SPG11 gene and further evidence for genetic heterogeneity. *Eur J Neurol.* 2009;16(1):121-6.

[19] Laura M, Pipis M, Rossor AM, Reilly MM. Charcot-Marie-Tooth disease and related disorders: an evolving landscape. *Curr Opin Neurol.* 2019;32(5):641-50.

[20] Pipis M, Rossor AM, Laura M, Reilly MM. Next-generation sequencing in Charcot-Marie-Tooth disease: opportunities and challenges. *Nat Rev Neurol.* 2019.

[21] Kalaydjieva L, Gresham D, Gooding R, Heather L, Baas F, de Jonge R, et al. N-myc downstream-regulated gene 1 is mutated in hereditary motor and sensory neuropathy-Lom. *Am J Hum Genet.* 2000;67(1):47-58.

[22] Brenner D, Weishaupt JH. Update on amyotrophic lateral sclerosis genetics. *Curr Opin Neurol.* 2019;32(5):735-9.

[23] Zou ZY, Zhou ZR, Che CH, Liu CY, He RL, Huang HP. Genetic epidemiology of amyotrophic lateral sclerosis: a systematic review and meta-analysis. *J Neurol Neurosurg Psychiatry.* 2017;88(7):540-9.

[24] Rosen DR, Siddique T, Patterson D, Figlewicz DA, Sapp P, Hentati A, et al. Mutations in Cu/Zn superoxide dismutase gene are associated with familial amyotrophic lateral sclerosis. *Nature.* 1993; 362(6415):59-62.

[25] Andersen PM, Nilsson P, Keranen ML, Forsgren L, Hagglund J, Karlsborg M, et al. Phenotypic heterogeneity in motor neuron disease

patients with CuZn-superoxide dismutase mutations in Scandinavia. *Brain*. 1997;120 (Pt 10):1723-37.

[26] Andersen PM. Amyotrophic lateral sclerosis associated with mutations in the CuZn superoxide dismutase gene. *Curr Neurol Neurosci Rep*. 2006;6(1):37-46.

[27] Zu JS, Deng HX, Lo TP, Mitsumoto H, Ahmed MS, Hung WY, et al. Exon 5 encoded domain is not required for the toxic function of mutant SOD1 but essential for the dismutase activity: identification and characterization of two new SOD1 mutations associated with familial amyotrophic lateral sclerosis. *Neurogenetics*. 1997;1(1):65-71.

In: Gene Mutations: Causes and Effects   ISBN: 978-1-53616-984-3
Editor: Helena M. Christoffersen   © 2020 Nova Science Publishers, Inc.

Chapter 3

ESR1 GENE AMPLIFICATION IN BREAST CANCERS IS AN EFFORT FOR DNA STABILIZATION AND A CONSEQUENTIAL TUMOR RESPONSE

Zsuzsanna Suba[*]

National Institute of Oncology, Department of Molecular Pathology,
Budapest, Hungary

ABSTRACT

The reported amplification of the estrogen receptor alpha gene (*ESR1*) in breast cancers initiated a broad and still ongoing scientific debate on the prevalence and clinical significance of this genetic alteration. The presented study analyses all conflicting data concerning the amplification of *ESR1* gene; its ambiguous prevalence in both untreated tumors and tumors either responsive or unresponsive to antiestrogen therapy. The fact will be highlighted that in healthy breast cells, the dynamism of genome stabilizer machinery may induce *ESR1* amplification when an emergency situation, such as estrogen deficiency requires a rapid compensatory upregulation of estrogen receptor (ER) expression and activation. In

[*]Corresponding Author's Email: subazdr@gmail.com.

contrast, in breast cancer cells, the feedback mechanism between *ESR1* gene and ERs exhibits failures attributed to various alterations of the genome stabilizer circuits. *ESR1* amplification in breast cancer cells may not be expected to show either a direct or indirect correlation with the aggressivity of tumors attributed to various disturbances of their regulatory processes. In antiestrogen treated breast cancers, basal failures of the genomic machinery are exaggerated via the artificial inhibition of the ER activation. The medical blockade of ERs is an emergency state even for tumor cells and a chaotic fight develops between the inhibition of ERs and the compensatory efforts for ER activation. When the medical ER blockade is successful, tumors exhibit unrestrained growth, whilst when the endogenous compensatory actions re-establish ER activation; tumors may show a clinical response. Abundant, reactivated ERs are capable of restoring the altered genomic machinery of tumor cells leading to a self directed apoptotic death. In conclusion, *ESR1* amplification is not an indicator of oncogenic adaptation in tumor cells, and it may not predict either the response or resistance of antiestrogen treated tumors.

Keywords: estrogen, antiestrogen, tamoxifen, aromatase inhibitor, estrogen receptor, ESR1 gene, EGF receptor, IGF1 receptor, gene amplification, antiestrogen resistance

INTRODUCTION

In 1990, Nembrot et al. reported an amplification of *ESR1 gene* occurring in breast cancers [1]. *ESR1 gene* encodes the estrogen receptor alpha (ER-alpha); a cellular receptor for estrogen hormones and its amplification may be in strong correlation with the overexpression of ER alpha protein in breast tumors.

ER alpha is activated by estrogen and exhibits a key role in the regulation of growth and differentiation of the mammary gland [2]. Excessive estrogen activation of ERs presumably initiates and drives an unrestrained proliferative activity in breast cells leading to the development of breast cancer [3]. About two thirds of breast cancers exhibit more or less ER alpha expression at the time of clinical diagnosis, which suggested that ER alpha protein may be a very important player in the development of mammary tumors and became a molecular target for tumor therapy [4].This postulation led to the introduction of antiestrogen therapy against breast cancer via either a blockade of liganded activation of ERs or an inhibition of estrogen synthesis [5,6]. However, antiestrogen therapies against breast cancer yielded fairly controversial results. More than a half of the targeted ER-positive breast cancers did not respond to the tamoxifen blockade of liganded ER activation [7]. Moreover, a long term antiestrogen therapy resulted in unresponsive or even rapidly growing tumors in the majority of ER-positive breast cancer cases [8].

In newly diagnosed, untreated breast cancers, an increased ER expression is the prerequisite of a good response to antiestrogen treatment leading to a better prognosis for the disease [9,10]. Unexpectedly, a similar overexpression of ERs was reported in tumor cells treated with either estrogens or antiestrogens [11,12]. In breast cancer cells, an overexpression of ERs through both estrogen and antiestrogen treatment initiates the upregulation of ER signaling and DNA stabilizer processes instead of a promotion of tumor growth [10]. Tumor responses to both estrogen and antiestrogen treatments suggest a fundamental regulatory capacity of ERs via either a direct or an indirect, compensatory activation [13].

Later on, in vitro experiments performed on tumor cell lines yielded highly controversial findings regarding the significance of ER-proteins and *ESR1* genes in the progression and regression of breast cancers. Experimental studies on breast cancer cell lines suggested that there are both ER dependent and ER independent mechanisms of breast carcinogenesis [14]. Interestingly, 5-10% of the ER-negative breast cancers have also shown sensitivity to tamoxifen treatment suggesting that there is a need of searching for alternative signaling pathways in tumor therapy independent of ER activation [15]. Moreover, in experimental studies, an inoculation of exogenous ER protein into ER-negative breast cancers induced a rapid tumor response to estrogen treatment [16,], indicating the pivotal role of estrogen activated ERs in DNA stabilization and a self directed tumor death [13].

After an initial enthusiasm, clinical experiences indicated that a long term antiestrogen therapy results in a secondary resistance in the majority of earlier responsive ER-positive breast cancers [8]. Tumors unresponsive to either tamoxifen treatment or long term estrogen deprivation (LTED) showed unrestrained growth, while exhibiting an overexpression of both ERs and growth factor receptors (GFRs) [17,18]. The abundance of ERs and GFRs in antiestrogen resistant tumors, mistakenly suggested that an excessive expression and crosstalk of these receptors is the key for tumor survival and the increasing aggressivity of tumors [19].

Gene amplification is defined as an increase in the copy number of certain genes in a cell. Gene amplification is presumably a critical mechanism for the oncogenic activation of genes [20,21] and it is regarded as a marker for oncogenic alterations [22,23]. Since ER protein expression in tumors, seemed to be the prerequisite of an effective response to antiestrogen therapy, the demonstration of *ESR1* amplification emerged as a candidate predictor for an optimal response of breast cancers to antiestrogen monotherapy [24].

However, the accounts of ESR1 amplification in breast cancers were controversial from the onset [25]. In 1991, Watts et al. reported an unexpected lower incidence of increased *ESR1* copy number in breast cancer while they used the same method as Nembrot et al. [26]. Later, various studies have published that *ESR1* amplification frequencies in breast tumors may range from 0% to 75% [25]. The wide range of diverging data strongly suggested that differences in tissue sampling and laboratory protocols may represent major difficulties in the analysis and estimation of *ESR1* amplification in breast cancers [27].

In antiestrogen treated breast cancers, the relevance of *ESR1* amplification has also been strongly disputed considering the experienced ambiguous data [28]. Predictive values for tumor responses associated with *ESR1* amplification were reported [24], whilst tumor resistance also was experienced in correlation with an increased *ESR1* copy number [29]. Prediction of a subsequent cancer development from precursor mammary lesions also was examined in correlation with displaying an amplification of *ESR1* gene [30].

The presented study analyses all conflicting data concerning activating mutations and amplification of *ESR1* gene found in untreated breast cancers and in tumors either responsive or unresponsive to antiestrogen therapy. The fact will be highlighted that in healthy cells the dynamism of genome stabilizer machinery will urge *ESR1* amplification when an emergency situation, such as estrogen deficiency, requires a rapid compensatory upregulation of ER expression. In contrast, in tumor cells, *ESR1* copy number and ER protein expression do not show a consequently direct correlation attributed to the defects of genomic machinery. In breast cancers, deregulations affecting different genomic pathways may result in a low *ESR1* copy number even in ER positive tumor cells. Conversely, in tumors, even an increased number of ESR1 copies may not be directly associated with a high expression and activity of ERs attributed to the various regulatory disorders occurring in both untreated and endocrine treated tumors.

In conclusion, high ER expression of an untreated tumor is a much better predictor for the curability of a cancer than *ESR1* amplification, as expression and activation of ERs are prerequisites for the upregulation of the DNA stabilizer circuit.

FUNDAMENTAL ROLES OF ER SIGNALING IN THE PHYSIOLOGY OF MAMMALIANS

ERs may act as a hub in the regulatory network, where all molecular signaling pathways are accumulated. Estrogen activated ERs as transcriptional factors drive the expression of appropriate estrogen regulated genes and their signals orchestrate all cellular functions [31].

Estrogens are synthesized by aromatase enzyme via converting androgens to estrogens. Estradiol (E2) is the most potent and abundant estrogen in the circulation, while estrone (E1) and estriol (E3) have weaker estrogenic activities. Two estrogen receptor isoforms, ER-alpha and ER-beta are members of the nuclear receptor superfamily and they exhibit strong crosstalk and interplay. ER-beta is mainly responsible for cellular enlargement, while the role of ER-alpha is crucial in regulating cell proliferation [32]. Both ER isoforms are mandatory regulators of cellular glucose uptake since cell growth and mitotic activity require an appropriate supply of fuel for increased metabolic processes [33,34]. Defective estrogen signaling induced by either estrogen deficiency or ER resistance leads to a deepening cellular insulin resistance [35,36].

ER-alpha and ER-beta proteins are expressed via transcriptional activities on *ESR1* and *ESR2* genes. Estrogen bound ERs may directly operate as ligand activated transcription factor proteins on the various promoter regions of target genes. ERs can also regulate gene expression through indirect binding to deoxyribonucleic acid (DNA) via interaction with transcription factor proteins. Moreover, cell membrane associated ERs may also confer non-genomic signaling cascades to estrogen dependent target genes. Unliganded activation of ERs may also be induced by mitogen-activated protein kinase (MAPK) or protein kinase B (Akt) pathways. Finally, genomic and non-genomic pathways of estrogen receptor signaling converge on the target genes [31].

The transcriptional activity of ERs partially results in the expression of protein coding ribonucleic acids (RNAs), whilst the vast majority of RNA transcripts are non-coding RNAs (ncRNAs) [37]. Protein coding RNA transcripts of ERs may define the synthesis of enzymes, receptors and further regulatory proteins. By contrast, ER-induced long non-coding RNA (lncRNA) transcripts are capable of promoting epigenetic gene modifications via their specific chromatin remodeling activities resulting in mutations on targeted genes [38]. lncRNAs are in close interrelationship with genome stabilizer proteins, such as p53, suggesting a pivotal role of these transcripts in the promotion of genome protecting mutations [37].

Estrogens are outstanding hormones exhibiting a strong, unique upregulative feedback mechanism with their own receptors. Both low and high estrogen levels drive the increased expression and transcriptional activity of ERs so as to restore or augment cellular ER signaling. In turn, both low and high ER expressions require upregulated estrogen synthesis for the improvement or augmentation of crucial estrogen signaling [39].

Upregulation of estrogen signaling displays a unique dichotomy via DNA stabilization, ensuring the survival or apoptosis and a safe proliferative activity of healthy cells, while inducing spontaneous death of malignant tumor cells [39]. Both protein coding and chromatin modifier RNA transcripts of ERs may have crucial roles in the genome stabilizer machinery [40].

ESTROGEN REGULATED GENES DRIVE ALL PHYSIOLOGICAL FUNCTIONS OF HEALTHY CELLS

Estrogen hormones activate ERs promoting the expression of estrogen regulated genes so as to initiate, complete and supervise the replication and recombination of DNA [31]. ER signaling has a crucial role in orchestrating all cellular functions including both metabolic processes and the rate of cell proliferation. There is a unique upregulative feedback mechanism between estrogens and their receptors. Both high and low estrogen levels induce an increased expression and transcriptional activity of ERs so as to restore or increase cellular ER signaling. In turn, both low and high ER expressions induce powerful estrogen synthesis for the improvement or appropriate augmentation of the crucial ER signaling [13, 39].

Estrogen activated ERs exhibit crucial anticancer effects [39]. Estrogen binding induces a liganded activation of ERs through their AF2 domain. Estrogen activated ERs induce the expression of copious ERs. Abundance of ERs enhances the expression of genome stabilizer proteins including BRCAs. Increased expression of genome stabilizer proteins activates aromatase enzyme synthesis and estrogen production providing abundant ligand for the extreme activation of plentiful ERs. This genome stabilizer circuit initiated by estrogen hormone ensures the upregulation of both ER signaling and DNA stabilization. The DNA protective circuit initiated by estrogen stimulation activates all physiologic functions of healthy cells, including both upregulation and downregulation of cell cycle, while inhibiting the survival possibility of cancer cells in a Janus-faced manner.

In conclusion, high estrogen concentrations are not obligate mediators for the excessive proliferation of either healthy or malignant cells, but rather they are principal regulators for ensuring cellular health and tumor death.

In an estrogen deficient milieu, the possibility of unliganded ER activation through the AF1 domain provides immense reserve capacities for the transient stabilization of genomic machinery [41]. Loss of estrogen endangers the liganded ER activation, while a prompt compensatory upregulation of unliganded ER activation may save the surveillance of the genomic machinery [10,42].

Estrogen hormones induce a balanced activation of both estrogen liganded and unliganded growth factor receptor (GFR) mediated transactivation functions of ERs [13]. Estrogen activated ERs regulate the expression and activation of growth factors and their membrane associated receptors promoting even the unliganded activation of ERs [43]. Experimental studies reveal a strong interplay between liganded and unliganded transcriptional activations of ERs [44]. In embryonic life, the ancient AF1 domain of ERs drives the development and differentiation. In adult men and women, the ligand dependent AF2 activation of ERs enjoys a conspicuous primacy; however, the AF1 domain also has a genome wide function even in adults, particularly in an emergency situation of estrogen deficiency [42].

Artificial inhibition of either liganded or unliganded ER activation provokes a strong compensatory upregulation of the unaffected domain [10]. A moderately defective function of the ligand dependent AF2 domain may be sufficiently restored by the activated AF1 domain. In contrast, a complete blockade of the superior AF2 domain may not be compensated even in a strongly estrogen rich milieu.

In healthy cells, ERs and *ESR* genes coding ER expressions are in strong crosstalk [13]. In case of decreased estrogen concentration, activated ER-alphas occupy the available ESR1 promoter regions inducing an increased expression of protein coding ER-alpha-mRNAs and leading to a self-generating increase in ER-alpha synthesis [39]. In emergency situations of regulatory disturbances, there is a further possibility for the endorsement of increased ER-alpha synthesis. Activated ER-alpha may occupy the promoter regions of long non-coding RNAs (lncRNAs), such as HOTAIR, which are ER responsive [45]. Increased expression of appropriate lncRNAs may provoke epigenetic changes on targeted *ESR1* promoter regions resulting in activating mutations and amplification of *ESR1* gene. These processes lead to overexpression and an increased E2 binding capacity of ERs in case of endangered ER signaling [13].

In conclusion, in healthy cells, *ESR1* gene amplification does not stand for an oncogenic alteration, but rather, it is an effort for the strengthening of genome stabilizer circuit through the upregulation of ER expression.

Estrogen exhibits antidiabetogenic effects. Estrogen activated ERs have beneficial effects on the energy metabolism and glucose homeostasis by means of several pathways [46]. Estrogen regulated genes drive all steps of insulin stimulated cellular glucose uptake from the insulin synthesis of β-cells in pancreatic islands to the expression of intracellular glucose transporters ensuring the fuel for all metabolic processes and genomic functions [33]. Estradiol treatment in healthy adipocytes promotes the nucleus-plasma membrane transport of ER alpha, increases AKT phosphorylation and glucose transporter 4 (GLUT4) expressions as well as GLUT4 translocation to the plasma membrane [47]. Consequently, defects in ER signaling attributed to either estrogen deficiency or ER resistance may lead to serious insulin resistance in correlation with the development of type 2 diabetes, cardiovascular diseases and malignancies [35]. In conclusion, in tumor cells, an estrogen induced activation of glucose uptake is not a fuel for cell growth and proliferation, but rather, it is a means for the restoration of DNA stability and self directed death.

Estrogen has anti-obesity effects. Estrogen activated ERs regulate the balance of lipolysis and lipogenesis in central adipose tissue, visceral organs and cardiovascular structures [34]. Central adipose tissue is a hub in the signaling network that controls and regulates visceral organs, heart and great arteries via an inter-tissue crosstalk. Defective estrogen signaling and/or a highly fat-rich diet induce an increased fat deposition in central adipocytes deteriorating their signaling functions [48]. Decreased expression of estrogen regulated genes is a key for the correlations between central obesity and obesity related comorbidities; type-2 diabetes, coronary heart disease and malignancies.

Estrogen has anti-atherogenic and anti-hypertensive effects. Healthy premenopausal women are typically protected from cardiovascular diseases and hypertension as compared with men. Conversely, diabetic young women and postmenopausal cases loose this protected state attributed to their estrogen resistance or fairly decreased bioavailable estradiol levels [49]. In premenopausal women, estrogen has crucial role in the maintenance of normal serum lipid levels [50]. Postmenopausal estrogen therapy reduces the risk of cardiovascular disease and this beneficial effect may be conferred by favorable changes in plasma lipid levels [51]. In postmenopausal women, estrogen treatment reduces the incidence of coronary atherosclerosis and myocardial infarction via an inhibition of vascular inflammation and increased nitric oxide formation [52]. Estradiol has a cardiovascular protective effect by its anti-hypertensive activity as well. Estrogen regulates the balance of renin-angiotensin system [53,54] and controls the synthesis of vasoconstrictor endothelin [55].

Estrogen regulates the balance of coagulation and fibrinolysis. In estrogen deficient postmenopausal women, a deregulation of hepatic glucose uptake and lipid metabolism leads to a non alcoholic liver steatosis. Steatosis of estrogen deficient liver is associated with an imbalance of the synthesis of procoagulant factors resulting in an increased level of factor VIII and a reduced level of protein C [56]. In cases with deficient estrogen signaling, an imbalance of coagulation and fibrinolysis might play a pivotal role in the development of thromboembolic complications, including cardiovascular diseases. Estrogen treatment increases the insulin sensitivity of liver [57] and improves the altered hepatic lipid metabolism in aged rats [58]. Postmenopausal hormone therapy improves hepatic glucose uptake, reduces hyperlipidemia and promotes a balanced synthesis of procoagulant factors [59].

ESTROGEN ACTIVATED ERs RECRUIT THE REMNANTS OF GENOME STABILIZER MACHINERY DRIVING A SELF DIRECTED DEATH IN TUMOR CELLS

In ER-positive tumor cells, an increased estrogen concentration results in a strong *upregulation of ER signaling* initiating a restoration of the genome stabilizer circuit and inducing a consequential self directed death [39]. In ER-negative breast cancer cells, estrogen treatment provokes tumor response after an exogenous ER inoculation [16].

In tumor cells, estradiol treatment *stimulates both liganded and unliganded ER activations.* In ER-positive breast cancer cell lines, estrogen treatment increases the expression and transcriptional activity of ERs as compared with those of untreated controls [11]. In breast cancer cells, estrogen treatment increased the expression of growth factor receptors (EGFR and HER2) upregulating even the unliganded activation of ERs [17]. Moreover, estradiol administration increases the activity of membrane associated phosphatidylinositol 3-kinase (PI 3-K)/Akt system [60]. In tumor cells, an estrogen induced activation of growth factor receptor (GFR) regulated pathways is not a survival technique but rather serves the improvement of DNA stabilization via an increased unliganded ER activation [10]. In conclusion, an amplified crosstalk between overexpressed ERs and GFRs serves as a means for restoring genomic stability in tumor cells so as to induce a tumor response.

In ER-positive breast cancer cell lines, treatment with four types of *estrogens provoked significant increases in ER-expression* as compared with the untreated controls [11]. Estrone, estradiol, estriol and estetrol were used as estrogen treatments. These results strongly suggest that in differentiated breast cancers, estrogen activated ERs increase the transcriptional activity on *ESR1* genes, while in turn; the high number of transcripts increases the translation of ER-alpha.

In breast cancer cells, estrogen administration usually induces an *amplification of ESR1 gene* at 6q25 locus upregulating ER protein synthesis [61]. During breast cancer "adaptation" a cluster of non coding RNAs was observed activating the *ESR1* locus [62]. Patients exhibiting *ESR1 gene* amplification in their breast tumors experienced a longer disease-free survival as compared with those without it [24]. These clinical experiences justify that in tumors an estrogen induced increased copy number of *ESR1* gene is not an oncogenic adaptation but rather it may help tumor responses through an abundant expression of ERs.

In tumor cells treated with estradiol, activated ERs mediate the transcriptional regulation and an *increased expression of lncRNAs*, including HOTAIR [45,63]. Increased expression of HOTAIR is associated with epigenetic changes in both *ESR1* and *BRCA1* genes, promoting ER-alpha expression, DNA stabilization and tumor regression [13]. Increased HOTAIR expression in the tumors of breast cancer cases was associated with lower risks of relapse and mortality as compared with those showing low HOTAIR expression in their tumors [64].

In breast cancer cells, estrogen activated ERs are capable of *increasing aromatase expression and estrogen synthesis*, which are essential for the increased liganded activation of ERs. Estradiol treatment elevated aromatase activity in a dose-dependent manner when ER-negative tumor cells were transfected with exogenous ER alpha [65]. In breast cancer cells, estradiol may increase the expression of aromatase enzyme through the activation of ER-alpha and upregulates aromatase activity as well by means of an enhanced tyrosine phosphorylation of the enzyme [66].

High *aromatase activity and an increased in situ estrogen concentration* were found at the invasive front of cancers, where interplay between the tumor and adjacent tissues may define the expansion or regression of cancer [67]. In breast cancer cases, a direct correlation was experienced between the aromatase activity of removed tumor samples and patient's survival time after surgery [68,69].

In MCF-7 tumor cell line, estrogen treatment induced an *increased expression of BRCA1 protein*. [70]. In turn, BRCA1 protein induces *ESR1*-gene activation resulting in an upregulation of ER-alpha mRNA expression and protein synthesis in breast cancer cell lines [71]. These observations justify that estrogen activated ER alpha and BRCA1 protein work in close partnership in the upregulation of genome stabilizer circuit promoting a self directed death of tumor cells [39].

In tumor cells, estradiol treatment *improves the insulin assisted glucose uptake*. In MCF-7 human breast cancer cells, estradiol has potentiating effects on insulin signaling via an enhanced expression of insulin receptor substrate-1 (IRS-1) [72]. In MCF-7 cell lines, estradiol enhances the entrance of glucose through the double lipid layer of cell membrane.

Estradiol treatment activates PI3K/Akt signaling pathway leading to a translocation of GLUT4 to the plasma membrane in an ER-alpha dependent manner [73]. These results reveal the mechanisms through which estrogen improves insulin assisted glucose uptake even in cancer cells providing energy for the restoration of DNA stability and promoting a self-directed apoptotic death [39].

INTERPLAY BETWEEN *ESR1* GENE COPY AND ER-ALPHA EXPRESSION ENSURES A BALANCE OF CELL PROLIFERATION IN HEALTHY BREASTS

Estrogen activated ERs are the primary initiators and organizers of the up-regulatory circle of genome stabilization in strong crosstalk with genome safeguarding proteins, and aromatase enzymes. The promoter regions of *ESR1*, *BRCA1*, and *CYP19* aromatase genes exhibit a triangular partnership for the harmonized regulation of the synthesis of ER-alpha, BRCA1 protein and aromatase enzyme [39].

Increased expression of *ESR1* gene is the main driver of genome stabilizer circuit in emergency situations attributed to either estrogen deficiency or ER-resistance.

The *transcriptional activities of ESR1 promoter regions* are initiated by activated ERs being responsible for the restoration of genome stabilizer machinery [13]. Activated ER-alpha assembles the most effective coactivators and occupies the available ESR1 promoter regions. The increased transcriptional activity of ER-alpha induces high expressions of protein coding ER-alpha-mRNAs and leads to a self-generating overexpression of ER-alpha. [39].

At the same time, a number of activated ER-alphas occupy the promoter regions of lncRNAs, e. g. HOTAIR, which are ER responsive [45]. Highly expressed lncRNAs are capable of provoking epigenetic changes on targeted *ESR1* promoter regions resulting in activating mutations. Newly formed activating mutations of *ESR1* genes induce an increased copy number and may lead to the overexpression and increased estrogen binding capacity of

ERs in an estrogen deficient milieu [62]. Abundant lncRNA transcripts of ERs are capable of inducing beneficial activating mutations on *BRCA1* promoters increasing the number of copies and BRCA protein expression [70,74] for the upregulation of DNA-stabilization.

The increasing expression of ER-alpha strongly upregulates aromatase synthesis as well and leads to increased estrogen production [39]. There are no literary data supporting the capacity of activated ER-alpha to occupy the *CYP19A* promoter region and induce directly an increased aromatase enzyme expression. It is likely that under physiologic conditions, ERs choose the safe circular pathway that induces increased aromatase expression through the activation of BRCA1 protein so as to achieve an appropriate estrogen synthesis.

On the contrary, it has been shown that in breast cancer cells lines, estradiol treatment can induce rapid increases in aromatase expression and estrogen synthesis by a nongenomic activation of ER-alpha via crosstalk with growth factor mediated pathways [62,66]. The quick upregulation of ER-alpha displays the existence of nongenomic, short autocrine loops between ER-alpha and aromatase enzyme synthesis providing rapid increase in estrogen production in emergency situations of malignancies.

The *transcriptional activities of the BRCA1 promoter regions* strengthen the stabilization of DNA. Activated ERs have the capacity to occupy the *BRCA1* promoter regions owing to the fact that *BRCA* genes are ER-alpha responsive [75]. Increased expressions of protein-coding BRCA1 mRNAs and elevated BRCA1 protein synthesis are driven by ER overexpression and high transcriptional activity, ensuring the adequate safeguarding of DNA-replication [39]. In turn, BRCA protein abundance promotes the expression of *ESR1*, the gene of ER-alpha [71].

Newly formed, abundant BRCA1 proteins are able to occupy the lncRNA promoters and also to increase the expression of lncRNAs. The abundance of lncRNAs may provoke beneficial epigenetic changes on *ESR1* promoters causing activating mutations and *ESR1* amplification resulting in an increased expression and liganded/unliganded activations of ER-alpha [76-78]. Further, lncRNA transcripts of BRCA1 may stimulate chromatin modifications on *CYP19* aromatase promoter genes and may induce highly increased aromatase synthesis and estrogen production [79,80]. Moreover, a BRCA1 protein stimulated expression of certain lncRNA transcripts confer activating mutations on *BRCA1* genes, ensuring an increased copy number and inducing an enhanced expression of DNA safeguarding BRCA1 proteins [13].

The *transcriptional activities of CYP19 aromatase promoter region* increase aromatase enzyme synthesis and estrogen production. Increased BRCA1 protein expression provides the opportunity of the considerable occupancy of *CYP19* aromatase promoter genes, which are responsive to BRCA1. Increased expression of the protein coding A450 mRNA results in upregulated synthesis of the aromatase enzyme capable of converting androgens to estrogens. Increased estrogen concentrations bind and activate abundant amounts of ER-alpha stimulating the upregulative circle of genome stabilization [39].

lncRNA promoter activation and increased lncRNA transcription by the BRCA1 protein may lead to activating mutation and amplification of the *CYP19* aromatase gene in order to increase aromatase synthesis and estrogen production [13]. In *BRCA1* mutation carriers, the liganded ER activation is weak, while BRCA1 protein activity confers a compensatory intensifying of estrogen synthesis through a selection of the appropriate *CYP19* aromatase promoter region [80].

UPREGULATIVE AND DOWN-REGULATIVE CROSSTALK BETWEEN ER-ALPHA AND BRCA1 IN PHYSIOLOGICAL AND MALIGNANT CELL PROLIFERATIONS

During a rapid physiological cell proliferation, as in case of pregnancy, the increased levels of estrogens activate available ER-alphas. Activated ER-alphas upregulate the expression of ER-alpha mRNA transcripts; inducing an abundant synthesis of ER-alpha protein [81]. Meanwhile, the high ER-alpha levels upregulate the expressions of protein coding BRCA1 mRNA transcripts and BRCA1-protein synthesis resulting in an increased safety of DNA stabilization [82,83]. In turn, high BRCA1-protein levels cause further upregulation in ER-alpha expression [84] and estrogen synthesis via an increased expression of both protein coding A450 mRNA transcripts and aromatase enzyme [80]. This upregulative circle ensures strong DNA-protection during the estrogen activated ER-determined rapid proliferation of maternal and fetal cells, whilst inducing apoptotic death in spontaneously initiated malignant cells [39].

In contrast, malignant cell proliferation manifests a self-repressing mutual down-regulation of the low and/or defective expressions of either ER-alpha or BRCA1-protein [39]. Mutagenic alteration or decreased expression of ER-alpha suppresses the expression of BRCA1 mRNA transcripts and BRCA1-protein synthesis; weakening appropriate DNA-safeguarding [83]. In turn, decreased or defective synthesis of the BRCA1-protein leads to down-regulation of both ER-alpha mRNA expression and ER-alpha synthesis and deteriorates ER-alpha signaling [85]. The down-regulative circle results in unrestrained proliferation of poorly differentiated tumor cells, which is attributable to the defect of ER signaling and the feeble control of DNA replication [39].

Moreover, the two key proteins; ER-alpha and BRCA1, are also capable of direct binding, thus mutually regulating their activities as transcriptional factors. Certain binding sites drive the upregulation of each other's transcriptional activity, while others may silence the transcriptional processes [84].

In sum, it may be established that in patients with cancer, the upregulation of ER-signaling by estradiol treatment may be the main method for a restoration of the physiologic circuit of cell proliferation and controlled DNA replication [86].

ALTERED CROSSTALK BETWEEN *ESR1* GENE COPY AND ER EXPRESSION IN UNTREATED BREAST CANCERS

In breast cancer cells, there are slight, moderate or great errors in the pathways of genome stabilizer circuit; resulting in different grades of differentiation and different failures in the expression of cellular receptors.

In untreated, newly diagnosed breast cancers, the higher the ER expression of tumors, the better is the prognosis of the disease [9]. This experience indicates that tumor cells express ERs providing possibilities for estrogen binding and ER activation so as to promote upregulation for ER signaling and DNA stabilization.

Highly ER positive breast cancers may exhibit spontaneous efforts for the self directed restoration of DNA stability indicated by a spontaneous *ESR1* gene amplification [39]. In these tumors, an upregulative crosstalk between *ESR1* copy number and ER expression may be observed promising a good tumor response to either estrogen or antiestrogen treatment [13]. Highly differentiated ER-positive breast cancer cells usually express an abundance of ERs asking for activation via estrogen binding [9]. In the background, activated ERs, as transcription factors promote an increased expression of newly formed ER proteins. At the same time, abundant, activated ERs increase the expression of appropriate lncRNAs so as to induce epigenetic changes in *ESR1* and resulting in activating mutations [13]. Abundant *ESR1* copies promote the further expression of ER proteins.

In moderately differentiated breast cancers with a lower expression of ERs, there are difficulties with the expression of ERs and/or with the activation of feedback mechanisms stimulating the amplification of *ESR1* gene [13]. In such tumors, either *ESR1* amplification or an extremely low copy number of *ESR1* gene may be observed. In these moderately differentiated tumors, there may be a compensatory increase in GFRs, including human epidermal growth factor receptor 2 (HER-2) providing possibilities for the increased unliganded activation of ERs [10]. For these tumors, an increased estrogen concentration is necessary to restore the ER activated amplification of *ESR1* gene and an increased genomic stability.

In ER negative tumors, usually a loss of *ESR1* copies may be observed depending on the location and type of regulatory disorders, while in certain cases, an increased *ESR1* copy number may also occur coupled with an apparent lack of ERs. The majority of these discrepant findings were attributed to technical and methodological reasons [25]. Nevertheless, *ESR1* amplification has been described in ER-alpha protein negative breast cancers, associated with a poor survival of the patients [87].

In apparently ER negative breast cancers, a compensatory overexpression of GFRs is a regular finding, which provides a possibility for an increased unliganded activation of scarcely occurring ERs [10]. In experimental studies, an inoculation of exogenous ERs into ER-negative tumors induced a rapid tumor response to estrogen treatment [16]. These results suggest that exogenous ER inoculation may be an effective therapeutic means against ER-negative breast cancers even in human practice.

Recent patent suggests a method for conversion of ER-negative breast cancers into ER-positive ones so as to increase antiestrogen sensitivity in poorly differentiated breast cancers [88]. This invention justifies the fact that in ER negative tumor cells a reactivation of ER signaling pathways plays crucial roles in the efficacy of treatment. Considering the pivotal regulatory role of activated ERs in the control of DNA stabilization, an estrogen stimulation of newly expressed ERs seems to be a more reasonable means to achieve tumor responses instead of an antiestrogen blockade of liganded ER activation [13].

Triple negative breast cancers (TNBCs) may be characterized by a poor histological differentiation and by a missing expression of receptors for estrogen, and progesterone as well as HER-2 [89]. These features of TNBCs indicate extensive regulatory disorders of estrogen signaling attributed to the failure of both liganded and unliganded activation of scarcely occurring ERs [9]. TNBC type tumors frequently exhibit mutation associated disorders in different genome stabilizer proteins, such as in BRCA and p53 [90,91] strongly inhibiting the circuit of genome stabilization.

In conclusion, in untreated breast cancers, the amount of activated ER expression is a much better prognostic indicator for the curability of tumors as compared with the fairly inconsistent *ESR1* amplification. Considering the numerous possibilities for the development of miscellaneous regulatory failures in tumors, neither a direct nor indirect correlation may be expected between ER expression and *ESR1* copy count.

ESR1 AMPLIFICATION SERVES AS AN EFFORT FOR DNA STABILIZATION IN EITHER ANTIESTROGEN RESPONSIVE OR RESISTANT TUMORS

Tamoxifen was developed as an anticancer agent working via an inhibition of the ligand dependent transactivation domain (AF2) of ERs in breast cancer cells [92]. The blockade of AF2 domain induces an extreme compensatory activation of AF1 domain provoking an increased expression of ERs, GFRs and aromatase enzyme in the genome stabilizer circuit [10]. Compensatory liganded and unliganded activation of abundant ERs may strongly increase the copy count of *ESR1* gene and may lead to a tumor response [13].

In antiestrogen responsive tumor cells, a strong compensatory upregulation of the earlier damaged ER signaling may lead to an apoptotic death, whilst in endocrine resistant tumors, an uncompensated, strong artificial ER blockade results in an unrestrained tumor growth.

In tamoxifen resistant breast cancer cell lines, an inhibition of the ligand dependent domain of ERs induced a compensatory overexpression of ER-alpha, which was evaluated as disturbing estrogen hypersensitivity and a key for antiestrogen resistance [12]. However, a similar overexpression of ERs in tumor cells treated with either estrogens [17] or antiestrogens [12] may be explained by the fundamental regulatory capacity and anticancer efficacy of activated ERs.

In reality, *in tamoxifen responsive tumors*, the compensatory upregulation of ER expression and intracrine estrogen synthesis provides possibilities for the restoration of ER signaling and for a self directed death of cancer cells [13]. Conversely, *in tamoxifen resistant tumors*, a long term endocrine treatment continuously stimulated the expression of ERs, while the growth of tumors was strongly progressive [93]. The incessant blockade of abundant ERs inhibited the feedback to *ESR1* genes resulting in a lower copy count than expected. Strikingly, tamoxifen resistant tumors, which were earlier stimulated by antiestrogen pretreatment, exhibited a marked tumor response to estradiol [93] attributed to a reactivation of abundant ERs and an increase in *ESR1* copy number.

In conclusion, a short term administration of tamoxifen may upregulate the compensatory ER expression of tumor cells leading to an apoptotic death. In contrast, an uncompensated tamoxifen-blockade on the AF2 domain of ERs promotes the proliferative capacity of tumor cells. However, an estradiol treatment of tamoxifen resistant tumors may restore DNA stabilization via an abundant expression and activation of newly formed ERs resulting in tumor regression [10].

Interestingly, 5-10% of the ER negative breast cancers have also shown sensitivity to tamoxifen treatment [15]. There is no need of searching for alternative signaling pathways independent of ER activation, as a few ERs may occur and work even in the apparently ER negative tumor cells.

In tamoxifen responsive tumor cells, expressions of membranous growth factor receptors (EGFR and HER2) were moderately increased as compared with detected expressions in control estrogen treated tumors. However, when tumors became antiestrogen resistant, highly increased expressions of both EGFR and HER2 were observed [17]. In tamoxifen treated tumor cells, an amplified crosstalk between upregulated ER and GFR pathways was regarded as a key for endocrine therapy resistance [94]. In reality, in tamoxifen responsive tumors, a moderate increase in GFR expression helps the compensatory unliganded activation of ERs leading to the restoration of ER activation. Conversely, in TAM resistant tumors, even a strongly increased expression of GFRs is not enough for the compensatory upregulation of ER expression and activation [10].

In breast cancer cells, estrogen withdrawal also induced a rapid increase in the unliganded activation of ERs through the utilization of GFR mediated MAP kinase and mTOR pathways provoking an adaptive estrogen hypersensitivity of tumor cells [18]. Long term estradiol deprivation (LTED) induced a strong upregulation of ER alpha expression in LTED resistant proliferative breast cancer cells, while an estrogen treatment induced their rapid apoptotic death [95]. In an estrogen deficient milieu, hypersensitivity to estrogen via a strong crosstalk between ERs and GFRs was regarded as a key mechanism for acquired antiestrogen resistance and tumor cell survival [96]. In reality, this adaptive estrogen hypersensitivity is not a survival technique of tumor cells, but rather it is an effort for the restoration of ER signaling and for self directed apoptotic death [10].

In tamoxifen treated tumor cells, an intracrine aromatase synthesis and increased estrogen concentrations provide further possibilities for the restoration of estrogen signaling and genomic stability [13]. In breast cancer cells, tamoxifen treatment increased the activity of aromatase promoter through an enhanced recruitment of c-fos/c-jun complex to AP-1 responsive elements located within the promoter region [66].

Estrogen treatment of breast cancer cell lines resistant to either long term estrogen deprivation (LTED-R) or tamoxifen (TAM-R) triggers an apoptotic death of tumor cells [19]. Considering the strong upregulation of both ER and GFR expressions in antiestrogen resistant tumors, estrogen seems to be an appropriate antiproliferative agent as it is capable of inducing a balanced activation of ERs through both liganded and non-liganded pathways [10]. In endocrine resistant tumor cells, compensatory increased expressions of ERs and GFRs as well as a strong upregulation of estrogen synthesis are efforts for the achievement of DNA stabilization counteracting the medical blockade of ER signaling. Estrogen treatment does not return antiestrogen resistant tumors to "antiestrogen responsiveness", but rather estrogen exerts its physiological antiproliferative effect overcoming the artificial blockade of ERs.

CONCLUSION

In healthy cells, both *ESR1* gene copy count and the expression of its protein products; ER-alphas, are increasing with the intensity of physiologic cell proliferation as ERs are the hubs of the network of DNA stabilizer signals. In contrast, in tumor cells, the unrestrained cell proliferation is not well controlled by the feedback mechanism between *ESR1* gene and ERs attributed to occurring different alterations in the genome stabilizer circuits. These disturbances clearly explain that *ESR1* amplification may not be in direct correlation with the development and aggressivity of breast cancer as it was strongly expected.

In antiestrogen treated breast cancers, basal failures of the genomic machinery are exaggerated with the artificial inhibition of liganded ER activation. The medical blockade of the chief regulator of genomic machinery is an emergency state even for tumor cells and a chaotic mixture develops between the ER inhibitor and compensatory activator processes. When an ER blockade is predominant, tumors exhibit an unrestrained proliferation, whilst in case of a successful compensatory upregulation of ER expression and activation, tumor regression will be the clinical response.

In conclusion, *ESR1* amplification may not be in direct correlation with either the response or resistance of tumors treated with antiestrogens.

REFERENCES

[1]   Nembrot M, Quintana B, Mordoh J. Estrogen receptor gene amplification is found in some estrogen receptor-positive human breast tumors. *Biochem Biophys Res Commun.* 1990; 166: 601-607.

[2]   Brisken C, O'Malley B. Hormone action in the mammary gland. *Cold Spring Harb Perspect Biol.* 2010; 2: a003178.

[3]   Russo J, Hu YF, Yang X, Russo IH. Developmental, cellular, and molecular basis of human breast cancer. *J Natl Cancer Inst Monogr.* 2000; (27): 17-37.

[4]   Allred DC. Issues and updates: evaluating estrogen receptor-alpha, progesterone receptor, and HER2 in breast cancer. *Mod Pathol.* 2010; 23 Suppl 2: S52-S59.

[5]   Jordan VC, Fritz NF, Langan-Fahey S, Thompson M, Tormey DC. Alteration of endocrine parameters in premenopausal women with breast cancer during long-term adjuvant therapy with tamoxifen as the single agent. *J Natl Cancer Inst.* 1991; 83(20): 1488-1491.

[6]   Buzdar AU, Jonat W, Howell A, et al. Anastrozole versus megestrol acetate in the treatment of postmenopausal women with advanced breast carcinoma: results of a survival update based on a combined analysis of data from two mature phase III trials. Arimidex Study Group. *Cancer.* 1998; 83(6): 1142-1152.

[7]   Hayes DF. Tamoxifen: Dr Jekyll and Mr Hyde? *J Natl Cancer Inst.* 2004; 96: 895-897.

[8]   Jordan VC. The new biology of estrogen-induced apoptosis applied to treat and prevent breast cancer. *Endocr Relat Cancer.* 2015; 22(1): 1-31.

[9]   Suba Z. Triple-negative breast cancer risk in women is defined by the defect of estrogen signaling: preventive and therapeutic implications. *OncoTargets Ther.* 2014; 7: 147-64.

[10]   Suba, Z. Amplified crosstalk between estrogen binding and GFR signaling mediated pathways of ER activation drives responses in tumors treated with endocrine disruptors. *Recent Pat Anticancer Drug Discov.* 2018; 13(4): 428-444.

[11]   Liu S, Ruan X, Schultz S, Neubauer H, Fehm T, Seeger H, et al. Oestetrol stimulates proliferation and oestrogen receptor expression in breast cancer cell lines: comparison of four oestrogens. *Eur J Contracept Reprod Health Care.* 2015; 20(1): 29-35.

[12]   Tolhurst RS, Thomas RS, Kyle FJ, Patel H, Periyasamy M, Photiou A, *et al.* Transient over-expression of estrogen receptor-α in breast cancer cells promotes cell survival and estrogen-independent growth. *Breast Cancer Res Treat.* 2011; 128(2): 357-68.

[13]   Suba Z. Activating mutations of ESR1, BRCA1 and CYP19 aromatase genes confer tumor response in breast cancers treated with antiestrogens. *Recent Pat Anticancer Drug Discov.* 2017; 12(2): 136-47.

[14]   Yue W, Yager JD, Wang JP, Jupe ER, Santen RJ. Estrogen receptor-dependent and independent mechanisms of breast cancer carcinogenesis. *Steroids.* 2013; 78: 161-170.

[15]   Manna S, Holz MK. Tamoxifen action in ER-negative breast cancer. *Signal Transduct Insights.* 2016; 10(5): 1-7.

[16]   Garcia M, Derocq D, Freiss G, Rochefort H. Activation of estrogen receptor transfected into a receptor-negative breast cancer cell line decreases the metastatic and invasive potential of the cells. *Proc Natl Acad Sci USA.* 1992; 89(23): 11538-42.

[17] Massarweh S, Osborne CK, Creighton CJ, Qin L, Tsimelzon A, Huang S, *et al.* Tamoxifen resistance in breast tumors is driven by growth factor receptor signaling with repression of classic estrogen receptor genomic function. *Cancer Res.* 2008; 68(3): 826-33.

[18] Santen RJ, Song RX, Masamura S, Yue W, Fan P, Sogon T, et al. Adaptation to estradiol deprivation causes up-regulation of growth factor pathways and hypersensitivity to estradiol in breast cancer cells. *Adv Exp Med Biol.* 2008; 630: 19-34.

[19] Mansouri S, Farahmand L, Hosseinzade A, Eslami-S Z, Majidzadeh-A K. Estrogen can restore Tamoxifen sensitivity in breast cancer cells amidst the complex network of resistance. *Biomed Pharmacother.* 2017; 93: 1320-5.

[20] Stratton MR, Campbell PJ, Futreal PA. The cancer genome. *Nature.* 2009; 458: 719-24.

[21] Santarius T, Shipley J, Brewer D, Stratton MR, Cooper CS. A census of amplified and overexpressed human cancer genes. *Nat Rev Cancer.* 2010; 10: 59-64.

[22] Sharma SV, Settleman J. Oncogene addiction: setting the stage for molecularly targeted cancer therapy. *Genes Dev.* 2007; 21: 3214-31.

[23] Comoglio PM, Giordano S, Trusolino L. Drug development of MET inhibitors: targeting oncogene addiction and expedience. *Nat Rev Drug Discov.* 2008; 7: 504-16.

[24] Tomita S, Zhang Z, Nakano M, Ibusuki M, Kawazoe T, Yamamoto Y, Iwase H. Estrogen receptor alpha gene ESR1 amplification may predict endocrine therapy responsiveness in breast cancer patients. *Cancer Sci.* 2009; 100: 1012-17.

[25] Holst F. Estrogen receptor alpha gene amplification in breast cancer: 25 years of debate. *World J Clin Oncol.* 2016; 7(2): 160-73.

[26] Watts CK, Handel ML, King RJ, Sutherland RL. Oestrogen receptor gene structure and function in breast cancer. *J Steroid Biochem Mol Biol.* 1992; 41: 529-536.

[27] Holst F, Moelans CB, Filipits M, Singer CF, Simon R, van Diest PJ. On the evidence for ESR1 amplification in breast cancer. *Nat Rev Cancer.* 2012; 12: 149.

[28] Lei JT, Gou X, Seker S, Ellis MJ. *ESR1* alterations and metastasis in estrogen receptor positive breast cancer. *J Cancer Metastasis Treat.* 2019; 5. pii: 38. Epub 2019 May 4.

[29] Nielsen KV, Ejlertsen B, Müller S, Møller S, Rasmussen BB, Balslev E, Lænkholm AV, Christiansen P, Mouridsen HT. Amplification of ESR1 may predict resistance to adjuvant tamoxifen in postmenopausal patients with hormone receptor positive breast cancer. *Breast Cancer Res Treat.* 2011; 127: 345-355.

[30] Soysal SD, Kilic IB, Regenbrecht CR, Schneider S, Muenst S, Kilic N, Güth U, Dietel M, Terracciano LM, Kilic E. Status of estrogen receptor 1 (ESR1) gene in mastopathy predicts subsequent development of breast cancer. *Breast Cancer Res Treat.* 2015; 151: 709-715.

[31] Maggi A. Liganded and unliganded activation of estrogen receptor and hormone replacement therapies. *Biochim Biophys Acta.* 2011; 1812(8): 1054-1060.

[32] Helguero LA, Faulds MH, Gustafsson JA, Haldosén LA. Estrogen receptors alfa (ERalpha) and beta (ERbeta) differentially regulate proliferation and apoptosis of the normal murine mammary epithelial cell line HC11. *Oncogene.* 2005; 24(44): 6605-16.

[33] Suba Z. Low estrogen exposure and/or defective estrogen signaling induces disturbances in glucose uptake and energy expenditure. *J Diabet Metab.* 2013; 4: 272-81.

[34] Suba Z. Circulatory estrogen level protects against breast cancer in obese women. *Recent Pat Anticancer Drug Discov.* 2013; 8(2): 154-67.

[35] Suba Z. Diverse pathomechanisms leading to the breakdown of cellular estrogen surveillance and breast cancer development: new therapeutic strategies. *Drug Design Devel Ther.* 2014; 8: 1381-90.

[36] Suba Z. Interplay between insulin resistance and estrogen deficiency as co-activators in carcinogenesis. *Pathol Oncol Res.* 2012; 18(2): 123-33.

[37] Baldassarre A, Andrea Masotti A. Long non-coding RNAs and p53 Regulation. *Int J Mol Sci.* 2012; 13(12): 16708-17.

[38] Gupta RA, Shah N, Wang KC, Kim J, Horlings HM, Wong DJ, et al. Long non-coding RNA HOTAIR reprograms chromatin state to promote cancer metastasis. *Nature*. 2010; 464(7291): 1071-6.

[39] Suba Z. DNA stabilization by the upregulation of estrogen signaling in BRCA gene mutation carriers. *Drug Des Devel Ther*. 2015; 9: 2663-75.

[40] Suba Z. Auto-regulative Circle of ER signaling drives the machinery of genome stabilization. *J Cancer Biol Res*. 2016; 4(4): 1089-97.

[41] Curtis SW, Washburn T, Sewall C, DiAugustine R, Lindzey J, Couse JF et al. Physiological coupling of growth factor and steroid receptor signaling pathways: estrogen receptor knockout mice lack estrogen-like response to epidermal growth factor. *Proc Natl Acad Sci USA*. 1996; 93(22): 12626-30.

[42] Caizzi L, Ferrero G, Cutrupi S, Cordero F, Ballaré C, Miano V, et al. Genome-wide activity of unliganded estrogen receptor-α in breast cancer cells. *Proc Natl Acad Sci USA*. 2014; 111(13): 4892-7.

[43] Hewitt SC, Li Y, Li L, Korach KS. Estrogen-mediated regulation of IGF1 transcription and uterine growth involves direct binding of estrogen receptor alpha to estrogen-responsive elements. *J Biol Chem*. 2010; 285(4): 2676-85.

[44] Arao Y, Hamilton KJ, Ray MK, Scott G, Mishina Y, Korach KS. Estrogen receptor α AF2 mutation results in antagonist reversal and reveals tissue selective function of estrogen receptor modulation. *Proc Natl Acad Sci USA*. 2011; 108(36): 14986-91.

[45] Bhan A, Mandal SS. Estradiol-Induced Transcriptional Regulation of Long Non-Coding RNA, HOTAIR. *Methods Mol Biol*. 2016; 1366: 395-412.

[46] Barros RP, Machado UF, Gustafsson JA. Estrogen receptors New players in diabetes mellitus. *Trends Mol Med*. 2006; 12(9): 425-31.

[47] Campello RS, Fátima LA, Barreto-Andrade JN, Lucas TF, Mori RC, Porto CS, Machado UF. Estradiol-induced regulation of GLUT4 in 3T3-L1 cells: involvement of ESR1 and AKT activation. *J Mol Endocrinol*. 2017; 59(3): 257-268.

[48] Suba Z. Crossroad between obesity and cancer: a defective signaling function of heavily lipid laden adipocytes (Online First). In: Crosstalk in Biological Processes. Ed: El-Esawi MA. *InTechOpen,* London, May 3rd 2019. doi: 10.5772/intechopen.85995

[49] Reckelhoff JF. Sex steroids cardiovascular disease and hypertension unanswered questions and some speculations. *Hypertension.* 2005; 45(2): 170-4.

[50] Jensen J, Nilas L, Christiansen C. Influence of menopause on serum lipids and lipoproteins. *Maturitas.*1990; 12(4): 321-31.

[51] Walsh BW, Schiff I, Rosner B, Greenberg L, Ravnikar V, Sacks FM. Effects of postmenopausal estrogen replacement on the concentrations and metabolism of plasma lipoproteins. *N Engl J Med.* 1991; 325(17): 1196-204.

[52] Meyer MR, Fredette NC, Howard TA, HuCh, Ramesh Ch, Daniel Ch, et al. G Protein-coupled Estrogen Receptor Protects from Atherosclerosis. *Sci Rep.* 2014; 4: 7564.

[53] Harrison-Bernard LM, Schulman IH, Raij L. Postovariectomy hypertension is linked to increased renal AT1 receptor and salt sensitivity. *Hypertension.* 2003; 42(6): 1157-63.

[54] Gallagher PE, Li P, Lenhart JR, Chappell MC, Brosnihan KB. Estrogen regulation of angiotensin-converting enzyme mRNA. *Hypertension.* 1999; 33(1 Pt 2): 323-8.

[55] Widder J, Pelzer T, vonPoser-Klein C, Hu K, Jazbutyte V, Fritzemeier KH, et al. Improvement of endothelial dysfunction by selective estrogen receptor-alpha stimulation in ovariectomized SHR. *Hypertension.* 2003; 42(5): 991-6.

[56] Tripodi A, Fracanzani AL, Primignani M, Chantarangkul V, Clerici M, Mannucci PM, et al. Procoagulant imbalance in patients with non-alcoholic fatty liver disease. *J Hepatol.* 2014; 61(1): 148-54.

[57] Bryzgalova G, Gao H, Ahren B, Zierath JR, Galuska D, Steiler TL, et al. Evidence that oestrogen receptor-alpha plays an important role in the regulation of glucose homeostasis in mice: Insulin sensitivity in the liver. *Diabetologia.* 2006; 49(3): 588-97.

[58] Hamden K, Carreau S, Ellouz F, Masmoudi H, El FA. Protective effect of 17beta-estradiol on oxidative stress and liver dysfunction in aged male rats. *J Physiol Biochem.* 2007; 63(3): 195-201.

[59] Salpeter SR, Walsh JM, Ormiston TM, Greyber E, Buckley NS, Salpeter EE. Meta-analysis effect of hormone-replacement therapy on components of the metabolic syndrome in postmenopausal women. *Diabetes Obes Metab.* 2006; 8(5): 538-54.

[60] Stoica GE, Franke TF, Moroni M, Mueller S, Morgan E, Iann MC, et al. Effect of estradiol on estrogen receptor-alpha gene expression and activity can be modulated by the ErbB2/PI 3-K/Akt pathway. *Oncogene.* 2003; 22(39): 7998-8011.

[61] Holst F, Stahl PR, Ruiz C, Hellwinkel O, Jehan Z, Wendland M, et al. Estrogen receptor alpha (ESR1) gene amplification is frequent in breast cancer. *Nat Genet.* 2007; 39(5): 655-60.

[62] Tomita S, Abdalla MO, Fujiwara S, Matsumori H, Maehara K, Ohkawa Y, et al. A cluster of noncoding RNAs activates the ESR1 locus during breast cancer adaptation. *Nat Commun.* 2015; 6: 6966.

[63] Zhang J, Zhang P, Wang L, Piao HL, Ma L. Long non-coding RNA HOTAIR in carcinogenesis and metastasis. *Acta Biochim Biophys Sin (Shanghai).* 2014; 46(1): 1-5.

[64] Lu L, Zhu G, Zhang C, Deng Q, Katsaros D, Mayne ST, et als. Association of large noncoding RNA HOTAIR expression and its downstream intergenic CpG island methylation with survival in breast cancer. *Breast Cancer Res Treat.* 2012; 136(3): 875-83.

[65] Kinoshita Y, Chen S. Induction of aromatase (CYP19) expression in breast cancer cells through a nongenomic action of estrogen receptor alpha. *Cancer Res.* 2003; 63(13): 3546-55.

[66] Catalano S, Giordano C, Panza S, Chemi F, Bonofiglio D, Lanzino M,et al. Tamoxifen through GPER upregulates aromatase expres-sion: a novel mechanism sustaining tamoxifen-resistant breast cancer cell growth. *Breast Cancer Res Treat.* 2014; 146(2): 273-85.

[67] Sasano H, Miki Y, Nagasaki S, Suzuki T. In situ estrogen production and its regulation in human breast carcinoma: From endocrinology to intracrinology. *Pathology International.* 2009; 59: 777-89.

[68] Evans TRJ, Rowlands MG, Silva MC, Law M, Coombes RC. Prognostic significance of aromatase and estrone sulfatase enzymes in human breast cancer. *J Steroid Biochem Mol Biol.* 1993; 44: (4-6): 583-7.

[69] Bollet MA, Savignoni A, De Koning L, Tran-Perennou C, Barbaroux C,Degeorges A, et al. Tumor aromatase expression as a prognostic factor for local control in young breast cancer patients after breast-conserving treatment. *Breast Cancer Res.* 2009; 11(4): R54.

[70] Kininis M, Chen BS, Diehl AG, Isaacs GD, Zhang T, Siepel AC, et al. Genomic analyses of transcription factor binding, histone acetylation, and gene expression. *Mol Cell Biol.* 2007; 27: 5090-104.

[71] Hosey AM, Gorski JJ, Murray MM, Quinn JE, Chung WY, Stewart GE. et al. Molecular basis for estrogen receptor alpha deficiency in BRCA1-linked breast cancer. *J Natl Cancer Inst.* 2007; 99:1683-94.

[72] Mauro L,Salerno M,Panno ML,Bellizzi D,Sisci D,Miglietta A, et al.Estradiol increases IRS-1 gene expression and insulin signaling in breast cancer cells. *Biochem Biophys Res Commun.* 2001; 288(3): 685-9.

[73] Garrido P, Morán J, Alonso A, González S, González C. 17β-estradiol activates glucose uptake via GLUT4 translocation and PI3K/Akt signaling pathway in MCF-7 cells. *Endocrinology.* 2013; 154(6): 1979-89.

[74] Jeffy BD, Hockings JK, Kemp MQ, Morgan SS, Hager JA, Jason Beliakoff J,et al. An estrogen receptor-alpha/p300 complex activates the BRCA-1 promoter at an AP-1 site that binds Jun/Fos transcription factors: repressive effects of p53 on BRCA-1 transcription. *Neoplasia.* 2005; 7: 873-82.

[75] Gorski JJ, Kennedy RD, Hosey AM, Harkin DP. The complex relationship between BRCA1 and ERalpha in hereditary breast cancer. *Clin Cancer Res.* 2009; 15(5): 1514-8.

[76] Wang C, Fan S, Li Z, Fu M, Rao M, Ma Y, et al. Cyclin D1 antagonizes BRCA1 repression of estrogen receptor alpha activity. *Cancer Res.* 2005; 65: 6557-67.

[77] Fan S, Wang J, Yuan R, et al. BRCA1 inhibition of estrogen receptor signaling in transfected cells. *Science.* 1999; 284: 1354-6.

[78] Zheng L, Annab LA, Afshari CA, Lee WH, Boyer TG. BRCA1 mediates ligand-independent transcriptional repression of the estrogen receptor. *Proc Natl Acad Sci. USA* 2001; 98: 9587-92.

[79] Simpson ER, Dowsett M. Aromatase and its inhibitors: significance for breast cancer therapy. *Recent Prog Horm Res.* 2002; 57: 317-338.

[80] Ghosh S, Lu Y, Katz A, Hu Y, Li R. Tumor suppressor BRCA1 inhibits a breast cancer-associated promoter of the aromatase gene (CYP19) in human adipose stromal cells. *Am J Physiol Endocrinol Metab.* 2007; 292: 246-252.

[81] Schumacher A, Costa SD, Zenclussen AC. Endocrine factors modulating immune responses in pregnancy. *Front Immunol.* 2014; 5: 196.

[82] Farmer H, McCabe N, Lord CJ, Tutt AN, Johnson DA, Richardson TB, et al.Targeting the DNA repair defect in BRCA mutant cells as a therapeutic strategy. *Nature.* 2005; 434: 917-21.

[83] Spillman M., Bowcock A. BRCA1 and BRCA2 mRNA levels are coordinately elevated in human breast cancer cells in response to estrogen. *Oncogene.* 13:1639-45, 1996.

[84] Fan S, Ma YX, Wang C, Yuan RQ, Meng Q, Wang JAet al. p300 Modulates the BRCA1 inhibition of estrogen receptor activity. *Cancer Res.* 2002; 62: 141-51.

[85] Russo J, Russo IH. Toward a unified concept of mammary carcinogenesis. Aldaz MC, Gould MN, McLachlan J, Slaga TJ. Eds. *Progress in Clinical and Biological Research.* New York. Wiley-Liss. 1997. 1-16.

[86] Suba Z. Causal Therapy of Breast Cancer Irrelevant of Age, Tumor Stage and ER-Status: Stimulation of Estrogen Signaling Coupled With Breast Conserving Surgery. *Recent Pat Anticancer Drug Discov.* 2016; 11(3): 254-66.

[87] Markiewicz A, Wełnicka-Jaśkiewicz M, Skokowski J, Jaśkiewicz J, Szade J, Jassem J, Zaczek AJ. Prognostic significance of ESR1

amplification and ESR1 PvuII, CYP2C19*2, UGT2B15*2 polymorphisms in breast cancer patients. *PLoS One.* 2013; 8: e72219.

[88] Eriksson U. Treatment of er-negative breast cancer with anpdgf-cc inhibitor and an anti-estrogen. WO2017081171A1 (2017).

[89] Davis AA, Kaklamani VG. Metabolic syndrome and triple-negative breast cancer: a new paradigm. *Int J Breast Cancer.* 2012; 2012: 809291. doi: 10.1155/2012/809291.

[90] Atchley DP, Albarracin CT, Lopez A, Valero V, Amos CI, Gonzalez-Angulo AM, Hortobagyi GN, Arun BK. Clinical and pathologic characteristics of patients with BRCA-positive and BRCA-negative breast cancer. *J Clin Oncol.* 2008; 26(26): 4282-8.

[91] Carey L, Winer E, Viale G, Cameron D, Gianni L.Triple-negative breast cancer: Disease entity or title of convenience? *Nat Rev Clin Oncol.* 2010; 7(12): 683-92.

[92] Osborne CK. Tamoxifen in the treatment of breast cancer. *N Engl J Med.* 1998; 339: 1609-18.

[93] Liu H, Lee ES, Gajdos C, Pearce ST, Chen B, Osipo C, Loweth J, McKian K, De Los Reyes A, Wing L, Jordan VC. Apoptotic action of 17beta-estradiol in raloxifene-resistant MCF-7 cells in vitro and in vivo. *J Natl Cancer Inst.* 2003; 95(21): 1586-97.

[94] Osborne CK, Shou J, Massarweh S, Schiff R. Crosstalk between estrogen receptor and growth factor receptor pathways as a cause for endocrine therapy resistance in breast cancer. *Clin Cancer Res.* 2005; 11(2 Pt 2): 865s-70s.

[95] Ariazi EA, Cunliffe HE, Lewis-Wambi JS, Slifker MJ, Willis AL, Ramos P, et al. Estrogen induces apoptosis in estrogen deprivation-resistant breast cancer through stress responses as identified by global gene expression across time. *PNAS.* 2011; 108 (47): 18879-86.

[96] Dowsett M, Martin LA, Smith I, Johnston S. Mechanisms of resistance to aromatase inhibitors. *J Steroid Biochem Mol Biol.* 2005; 95(1-5): 167-72.

INDEX

D

E

DNA: Background, Laws and Backlog of Evidence

Editor: Tomáš Koláček

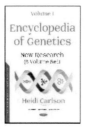

Series: Genetics – Research and Issues

Book Description: Deoxyribonucleic acid, or DNA, is the fundamental building block for an individual's entire genetic makeup. DNA is a powerful tool for law enforcement investigations because each person's DNA is different from that of every other individual (except for identical twins).

Hardcover ISBN: 978-1-53616-117-5
Retail Price: $160

Encyclopedia of Genetics: New Research (8 Volume Set)

Editor: Heidi Carlson

Series: Genetics – Research and Issues

Book Description: This 8 volume encyclopedia set presents important research on genetics. Some of the topics discussed herein include the speciation of Arabian gazelles, tau alternative splicing in Alzheimer's disease, Cornelia de Lange syndrome and autosomal dominant polycystic kidney disease.

Hardcover ISBN: 978-1-53614-451-2
Retail Price: $1,380

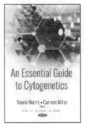